Nerve and Muscle

Written with undergraduate students in mind, the new edition of this classic textbook provides a compact introduction to the physiology of nerve and muscle. It gives a straightforward account of the fundamentals of this subject, accompanied by some of the experimental evidence upon which this understanding is based.

It first explores the nature of nerve impulses, clarifying their underlying mechanisms in terms of ion flow through molecular channels in the cell membrane. There then follows an account of the synaptic transmission processes by which one excitable cell influences activity in another. Finally, the emphasis turns to the consequences of excitable activity in the form of the activation of contraction in skeletal, cardiac and smooth muscle, highlighting the relationships between cellular structure and function.

This fourth edition includes new material on the molecular nature of ion channels, the activation of skeletal muscle and the function of cardiac and smooth muscle, reflecting exciting new developments in these rapidly growing fields.

Richard D. Keynes was Emeritus Professor of Physiology at the University of Cambridge.

David J. Aidley was Senior Fellow in the School of Biological Sciences at the University of East Anglia, Norwich.

Christopher L.-H. Huang is Professor of Cell Physiology at the University of Cambridge.

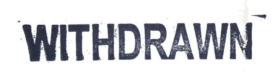

Nerve and Muscle

Fourth Edition

Richard D. Keynes
*Emeritus Professor of Physiology in the
University of Cambridge and
Fellow of Churchill College*

David J. Aidley
*Senior Fellow, Biological Sciences, University of
East Anglia, Norwich*

and

Christopher L.-H. Huang
*Professor of Cell Physiology in the University of
Cambridge and Fellow of Murray Edwards College*

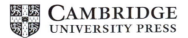
CAMBRIDGE
UNIVERSITY PRESS

CAMBRIDGE UNIVERSITY PRESS
Cambridge, New York, Melbourne, Madrid, Cape Town, Singapore,
São Paulo, Delhi, Dubai, Tokyo, Mexico City

Cambridge University Press
The Edinburgh Building, Cambridge CB2 8RU, UK

Published in the United States of America by
Cambridge University Press, New York

www.cambridge.org
Information on this title: www.cambridge.org/9780521519557

First published 1981
Second edition 1991
Third edition 2001
Fourth edition 2011

Printed in the United Kingdom at the University Press, Cambridge

A catalogue record for this publication is available from the British Library

Library of Congress Cataloging in Publication data
Keynes, R. D.
   Nerve and muscle / Richard D. Keynes, David J. Aidley,
   Christopher L.-H. Huang. – 4th ed.
      p.   cm.
   Includes bibliographical references and index.
   ISBN 978-0-521-51955-7 – ISBN 978-0-521-73742-5 (pbk.)
   1. Myoneural junction.   2. Neuromuscular transmission.   3. Muscle
   contraction.   I. Aidley, David J.   II. Huang, Christopher L.-H.   III. Title.
   QP321.K44 2011
   573.7′528–dc22   2010034899

ISBN 978-0-521-51955-7 Hardback
ISBN 978-0-521-73742-5 Paperback

Contents

Preface

Initiation of movement, whether in the form of voluntary action by skeletal muscle, or the contraction of cardiac or smooth muscle, is the clearest observable physiological manifestation of animal life. It inevitably involves activation of contractile tissue initiated or modulated by altered activity in its nerve supply. An appreciation of the function of nerve and muscle, and of the relationships between them is thus fundamental to our understanding of the function of the human body.

This book provides an introductory account of this important aspect of physiology, in a form suitable for students taking university courses in physiology, cell biology or medicine. It seeks to give a straightforward account of the fundamentals in this area, whilst including some of the experimental evidence upon which our conclusions are based.

This fourth edition includes new material reflecting the exciting discoveries concerning the ion channels involved in electrical activity, the activation of skeletal muscle and the function of cardiac and smooth muscle, reflecting important new developments made in these rapidly growing fields. We are grateful for expert advice and specialist comments from Drs. James Fraser, Ian Sabir and Juliet Usher-Smith, Physiological Laboratory, Cambridge, and Thomas Pedersen, Department of Physiology, University of Aarhus, and continue to benefit from the insight and wisdom left us by the late David Aidley, in these revisions.

R. D. Keynes
C. L.-H. Huang
Cambridge, Lent Term, 2010

Publishers' Note

Richard Keynes died peacefully at home while the proofs for this current edition were in preparation, ending a long and successful career as a university academic, in the international promotion of science, and as a cell physiologist. His scientific contributions had begun with radioactive tracer measurements of transmembrane movements of ions during activity in excitable cells, and the maintenance of their cellular concentrations through active transport processes. They went on to classic physiological studies of voltage generation in the electric eel, and measurements of thermal and optical changes in nerve and electric organs, and ion transport through secretory epithelia. They later returned to his original interests in the biophysical properties of nerve membranes through explorations of the molecular mechanisms underlying sodium-channel function by direct measurement and exploration of the gating currents associated with their activation. *Nerve and Muscle* (with David Aidley) first appeared in 1981. This current edition contains the last academic writings from his pen. We join his many friends in lamenting his death and extending our condolences to his wife Anne and their family.

1

Structural organization of the nervous system

1.1 | Nervous systems

One of the characteristics of higher animals is their possession of a more or less elaborate system for the rapid transfer of information through the body in the form of electrical signals, or nervous impulses. At the bottom of the evolutionary scale, the nervous system of some primitive invertebrates consists simply of an interconnected network of undifferentiated nerve cells. The next step in complexity is the division of the system into *sensory* nerves responsible for gathering incoming information, and *motor* nerves responsible for bringing about an appropriate response. The nerve cell bodies are grouped together to form *ganglia*. Specialized receptor organs are developed to detect every kind of change in the external and internal environment; and likewise there are various types of effector organ formed by muscles and glands, to which the outgoing instructions are channelled. In invertebrates, the ganglia which serve to link the inputs and outputs remain to some extent anatomically separate, but in vertebrates the bulk of the nerve cell bodies are collected together in the *central nervous system*. The *peripheral nervous system* thus consists of *afferent* sensory nerves conveying information to the central nervous system, and *efferent* motor nerves conveying instructions from it. Within the central nervous system, the different pathways are connected up by large numbers of *interneurons* which have an integrative function.

Certain ganglia involved in internal homeostasis remain outside the central nervous system. Together with the preganglionic nerve trunks leading to them, and the post-ganglionic fibres arising from them, which innervate smooth muscle and gland cells in the animal's viscera and elsewhere, they constitute the *autonomic nervous system*. The preganglionic autonomic fibres leave the central nervous system in two distinct outflows. Those in the cranial and sacral nerves form the *parasympathetic* division of the autonomic system, while those coming from the thoracic and lumbar segments of the spinal cord form the *sympathetic* division.

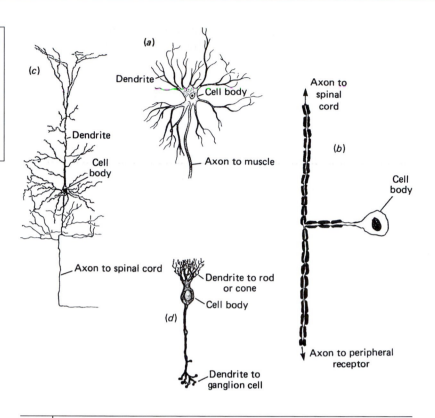

Figure 1.1 Schematic diagrams (not to scale) of the structure of: (*a*) a spinal motoneuron; (*b*) a spinal sensory neuron; (*c*) a pyramidal cell from the motor cortex of the brain; (*d*) a bipolar neuron in the vertebrate retina. (Adapted from Nichols *et al.*, 2001.)

1.2 | The anatomy of a neuron

Each neuron has a cell body in which its nucleus is located, and a number of processes or *dendrites* (Figure 1.1). One process, usually much longer than the rest, is the *axon* or nerve fibre which carries the outgoing impulses. The incoming signals from other neurons are passed on at junctional regions known as *synapses* scattered over the cell body and dendrites, but discussion of their structure and of the special mechanisms involved in synaptic transmission will be deferred to Chapters 7 and 8. At this stage we are concerned only with the properties of peripheral nerves, and need not concern ourselves further with the cell body, for although its intactness is essential in the long term to maintain the axon in working order, it does not actually play a direct role in the conduction of impulses. A nerve can continue to function for quite a while after being severed from its cell body, and electrophysiologists would have a hard time if this were not the case.

1.3 | Non-myelinated nerve fibres

Vertebrates have two main types of nerve fibre, the larger fast-conducting axons, 1 to 25 μm in diameter, being *myelinated*, and the small slowly conducting ones (under 1 μm) being *non-myelinated*.

Most of the fibres of the autonomic system are non-myelinated, as are peripheral sensory fibres subserving sensations like pain and temperature, where a rapid response is not required. Almost all invertebrates are equipped exclusively with non-myelinated fibres, but where rapid conduction is called for, their diameter may be as much as 500 or even 1000 μm. As will be seen in subsequent chapters, the giant axons of invertebrates have been extensively exploited in experiments on the mechanism of conduction of the nervous impulse. The major advances made in electrophysiology during the last 50 years have very often depended heavily on the technical possibilities opened up by the size of the squid giant axon.

All nerve fibres consist essentially of a long cylinder of cytoplasm, the *axoplasm*, surrounded by an electrically excitable *nerve membrane*. Now the electrical resistance of the axoplasm is fairly low, by virtue of the K^+ and other ions that are present in appreciable concentrations, while that of the membrane is relatively high, and the salt-containing body fluids outside the membrane are again good conductors of electricity. Nerve fibres therefore have a structure analogous to that of a shielded electric cable, with a central conducting core surrounded by insulation, outside which is another conducting layer. Many features of the behaviour of nerve fibres depend intimately on their *cable structure*.

The layer analogous with the insulation of the cable does not, however, consist solely of the high-resistance nerve membrane, owing to the presence of *Schwann cells*, which are wrapped around the *axis cylinder* in a manner which varies in the different types of nerve fibre. In the case of the olfactory nerve (Figure 1.2), a single Schwann cell serves as a multi-channel supporting structure enveloping a short stretch of 30 or more tiny axons. Elsewhere, each axon may be more or less closely associated with a Schwann cell of its own, some being deeply embedded within the Schwann cell, and others almost uncovered. In general, as in the example shown in Figure 1.3, each Schwann cell supports a small group of up to half a dozen axons. In the large invertebrate axons (Figure 1.4) the ratio is reversed, the whole surface of the axon being covered with a mosaic of many Schwann cells interdigitated with one another to form a layer several cells thick. In all non-myelinated nerves, both large and small, the axon membrane is separated from the Schwann cell membrane by a space about 10 nm wide, sometimes referred to by anatomists as the *mesaxon*. This space is in free communication with the main extracellular space of the tissue, and provides a relatively uniform pathway for the electric currents which flow during the passage of an impulse. However, it is a pathway that can be quite tortuous, so that ions which move out through the axon membrane in the course of an impulse are prevented from mixing quickly with extracellular ions, and may temporarily pile up outside, thus contributing to the *after-potential* (see Section 6.5). Nevertheless, for the immediate

Figure 1.2 Electron micrograph of a section through the olfactory nerve of a pike, showing a bundle of non-myelinated nerve fibres partially separated from other bundles by the basement membrane *B*. The mean diameter of the fibres is 0.2 μm, except where they are swollen by the presence of a mitochondrion (*M*). Magnification 54 800 ×. (Reproduced by courtesy of Prof. E. Weibel.)

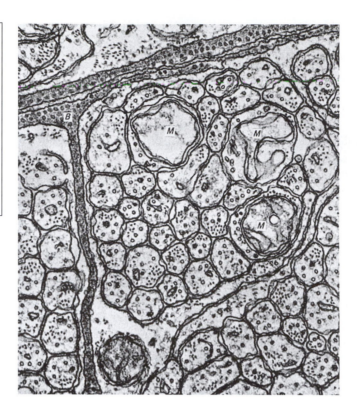

purpose of describing the way in which nerve impulses are propagated, non-myelinated fibres may be regarded as having a uniformly low external electrical resistance between different points on the outside of the membrane.

1.4 | Myelinated nerve fibres

In the myelinated nerve fibres of vertebrates, the excitable membrane is insulated electrically by the presence of the *myelin sheath* everywhere except at the *node of Ranvier* (Figures 1.5, 1.6, 1.7). In the case of peripheral nerves, each stretch of myelin is laid down by a Schwann cell that repeatedly envelops the axis cylinder with many concentric layers of cell membrane (Figure 1.7); in the central nervous system, it is the cells known as *oligodendroglia* that lay down the myelin. All cell membranes consist of a double layer of lipid molecules with which some proteins are associated (see Section 3.1), forming a structure that after appropriate staining appears under the electron microscope as a pair of dark lines 2.5 nm across, separated by a 2.5 nm gap. In an adult myelinated fibre, the adjacent layers of Schwann cell membrane are partly fused together at their cytoplasmic surface, and the overall repeat distance of the double membrane as determined by X-ray diffraction is 17 nm. For a nerve fibre whose outside diameter is 10 μm, each stretch of myelin is

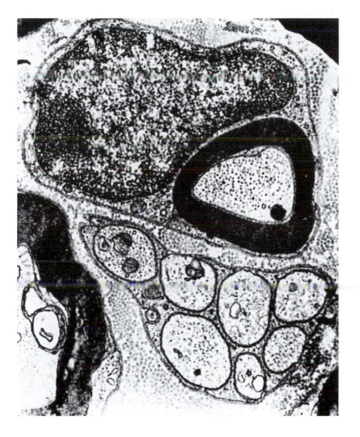

Figure 1.3 Electron micrograph of a cross-section through a mammalian nerve showing non-myelinated fibres with their supporting Schwann cells and some small myelinated fibres. (Reproduced by courtesy of Professor J. D. Robertson.)

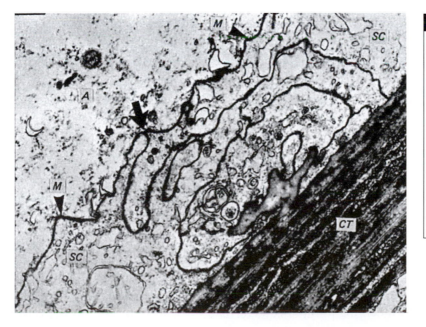

Figure 1.4 Electron micrograph of the surface of a squid giant axon, showing the axoplasm (A), Schwann cell layer (SC) and connective tissue sheath (CT). Ions crossing the excitable membrane (M, arrowheads) must diffuse laterally to the junction between neighbouring Schwann cells marked with an arrow, and thence along the gap between the cells into the external medium. Magnification 22 600 ×. (Reproduced by courtesy of Dr F. B. P. Wooding.)

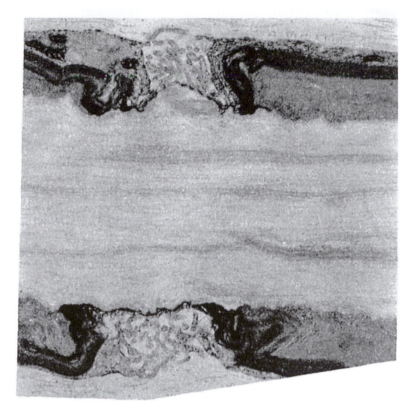

Figure 1.5 Electron micrograph of a node of Ranvier in a single fibre dissected from a frog nerve. (Reproduced by courtesy of Professor R. Stämpfli.)

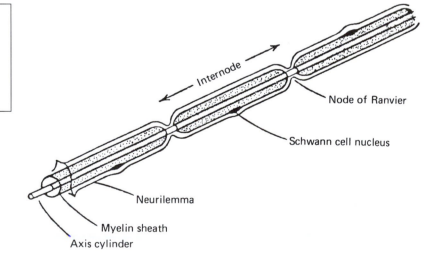

Figure 1.6 Schematic diagram of the structure of a vertebrate myelinated nerve fibre. The distance between neighbouring nodes is actually about 40 times greater relative to the fibre diameter than is shown here.

Internode

Node of Ranvier

Schwann cell nucleus

Neurilemma

Myelin sheath

Axis cylinder

about 1000 μm long and 1.3 μm thick, so that the myelin is built up of some 75 double layers of Schwann cell membrane. In larger fibres, the internodal distance, the thickness of the myelin and hence the number of layers, are all proportionately greater. Since myelin has a much higher lipid content than cytoplasm, it also has a greater

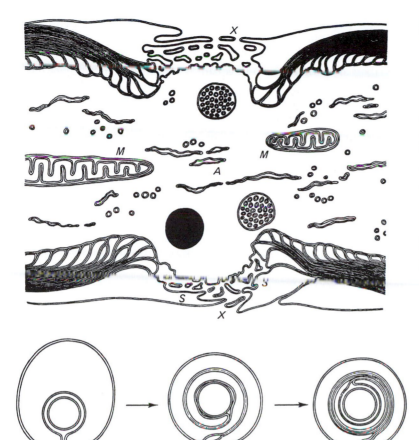

Figure 1.7 Drawing of a node of Ranvier made from an electron micrograph. The axis cylinder *A* is continuous through the node; the axoplasm contains mitochondria (*M*) and other organelles. The myelin sheath, laid down as shown below by repeated envelopment of the axon by the Schwann cell on either side of the node, is discontinuous, leaving a narrow gap *X*, where the excitable membrane is accessible to the outside. Small tongues of Schwann cell cytoplasm (*S*) project into the gap, but do not close it entirely. (From Robertson, 1960.)

refractive index, and in unstained preparations has a characteristic glistening white appearance. This accounts for the name given to the peripheral *white matter* of the spinal cord, consisting of columns of myelinated nerve fibres, as contrasted with the central core of *grey matter*, which is mainly nerve cell bodies and supporting tissue. It also accounts for the difference between the white and grey rami of the autonomic system, containing respectively small myelinated nerve fibres and non-myelinated fibres.

At the node of Ranvier, the closely packed layers of Schwann cells terminate on either side as a series of small tongues of cyto-plasm (Figure 1.7), leaving a gap about 1 μm in width where there is no obstacle between the axon membrane and the extra-cellular fluid. The external electrical resistance between neighbouring nodes of Ranvier is therefore relatively low, whereas the resistance between any two points on the internodal stretch of membrane is high because of the insulating effect of the myelin. The difference between the nodes and internodes in accessibility to the external medium is the basis for the *saltatory* mechanism of conduction in myelinated fibres (see Section 6.2), which enables them to conduct impulses some 50 times faster than a non-myelinated fibre of the same overall diameter. Nerves may branch many times before terminating, and the branches always arise at nodes.

In peripheral myelinated nerves the whole axon is usually described as being covered by a thin, apparently structureless basement membrane, the *neurilemma*. The nuclei of the Schwann cells are to be found just beneath the neurilemma, at the midpoint of each internode. The fibrous connective tissue which separates individual fibres is known as the *endoneurium*. The fibres are bound together in bundles by the *perineurium*, and the several bundles which in turn form a whole nerve trunk are surrounded by the *epineurium*. The connective tissue sheaths in which the bundles of nerve fibres are wrapped also contain continuous sheets of cells which prevent extracellular ions in the spaces between the fibres from mixing freely with those outside the nerve trunk. The barrier to free diffusion offered by the sheath is probably responsible for some of the experimental discrepancies between the behaviour of fibres in an intact nerve and that of isolated single nerve fibres. The nerve fibres within the brain and spinal cord are packed together very closely, and are usually said to lack a neurilemma. The individual fibres are difficult to tease apart, and the nodes of Ranvier are less easily demonstrated than in peripheral nerves by such histological techniques as staining with $AgNO_3$.

Resting and action potentials

2.1 | Electrophysiological recording methods

Although the nervous impulse is accompanied by effects that can under especially favourable conditions be detected with radioactive tracers, or by optical and thermal techniques, electrical recording methods normally provide much the most sensitive and convenient approach. A brief account is therefore necessary of some of the technical problems that arise in making good measurements both of steady electrical potentials and rapidly changing ones.

In order to record the potential difference between two points, electrodes connected to a suitable amplifier and recording system must be placed at each of them. If the investigation is only concerned with action potentials, fine platinum or tungsten wires can serve as electrodes, but any bare metal surface has the disadvantage of becoming *polarized* by the passage of electric current into or out of the solution with which it is in contact. When, therefore, the magnitude of the steady potential at the electrode tip is to be measured, non-polarizable or reversible electrodes must be used, for which the unavoidable *contact potential* between the metal and the solution is both small and constant. The simplest type of reversible electrode is provided by coating a silver wire electrolytically with AgCl, but for the most accurate measurements calomel ($Hg/HgCl_2$) half-cells are best employed.

When the potential inside a cell is to be recorded, the electrode has to be very well insulated except at its tip, and so fine that it can penetrate the cell membrane with a minimum of damage and without giving rise to electrical leaks. The earliest intracellular recordings were actually made by pushing a glass capillary 50 μm in diameter longitudinally down a 500 μm squid axon through a cannula tied into the cut end (Figure 2.1a), but this method cannot be applied universally. For tackling cells other than giant axons, glass microelectrodes are made by taking hard glass tubing about 2 mm in diameter and drawing down a short section to produce a tapered micropipette less than 0.5 μm across at the tip (Figure 2.1b). The

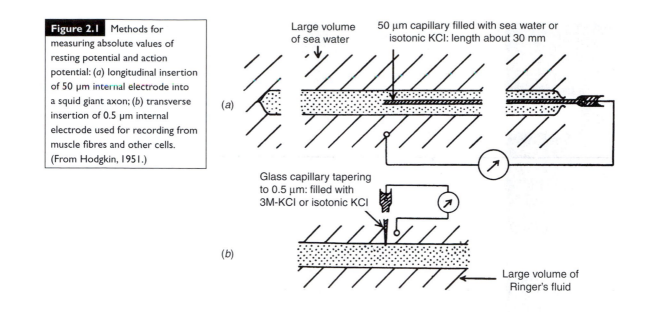

Figure 2.1 Methods for measuring absolute values of resting potential and action potential: (*a*) longitudinal insertion of 50 μm internal electrode into a squid giant axon; (*b*) transverse insertion of 0.5 μm internal electrode used for recording from muscle fibres and other cells. (From Hodgkin, 1951.)

microelectrode is then filled with 3 M KCl, and an Ag/AgCl electrode is inserted at the wide end. With various refinements, microelectrodes of this type have been used for direct measurement of the membrane potential not only in single neurons, but also in many other types of cell.

The potentials to be measured in electrophysiological experiments range from 150 mV down to a few μV, and in order to record them faithfully the frequency response of the system needs to be flat from zero to about 50 kilohertz (1 Hertz = 1 cycle/s). In addition to providing the necessary degree of amplification, the amplifier must have a very high input resistance, and must generate as little electrical noise as possible in the absence of an input signal. Now that high-quality solid-state operational amplifiers are readily available, there is no difficulty in meeting these requirements. The output is usually displayed on a cathode-ray oscilloscope, ideally fitted with a storage tube so that the details of the signals can be examined at leisure. To obtain a permanent record, the picture on the screen may be photographed. Direct-writing recorders yielding a continuous record on a reel of paper are convenient for some purposes, but cannot generally follow high frequencies well enough to reproduce individual action potentials with acceptable fidelity. A recent development for experiments involving close examination of the time course of the signals is to convert them into digital form, and to use an online computer both for storage and analysis of the data (Figures 4.12, 4.13).

A technique that since its introduction by Hodgkin and Huxley in 1949 has played an ever more important role in investigations of the mechanism of excitability in nerve and muscle is *voltage-clamping*. Its object, as explained in Section 4.3, is to enable the experimenter to explore the relationship between the potential difference across the membrane and its permeability to Na⁺ and K⁺ ions, by

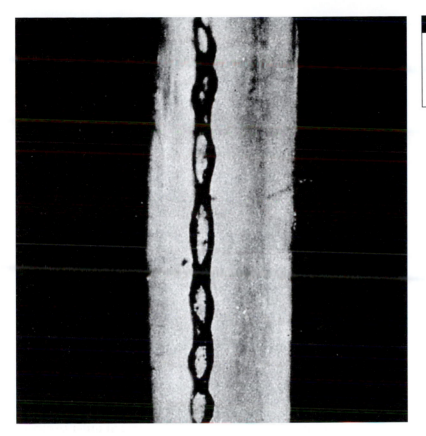

Figure 2.2 A squid giant axon into which a double spiral electrode has been inserted, photographed under a polarizing microscope. Its diameter was 700 µm.

clamping the membrane potential at a predetermined level and then measuring the changes in membrane current resulting from imposition of a voltage step. As shown diagrammatically in Figure 4.6, it necessitates the introduction of two electrodes into the axon, one of which monitors the membrane potential in the usual way, while the other is connected to the output of a feedback amplifier that produces just sufficient current to hold the potential at the desired value. The internal electrode system used by Hodgkin and Huxley was a double spiral of chloride-coated silver wire wound on a fine glass rod (Figure 2.2), but others have used a glass microcapillary as the voltage electrode, to which is glued an Ag/AgCl or platinized platinum wire to carry the current. In order to voltage-clamp the node of Ranvier in a single myelinated fibre dissected from a frog nerve, an entirely different electrode system is required, but the basic principle is the same.

2.2 | Intracellular recording of the membrane potential

When for the first time Hodgkin and Huxley measured the absolute magnitude of the electrical potential in a living cell by introducing

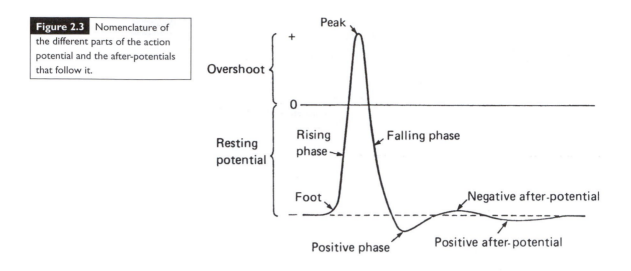

Figure 2.3 Nomenclature of the different parts of the action potential and the after-potentials that follow it.

a 50 µm capillary electrode into a squid giant axon, they found that when the tip of the electrode was far enough from the cut end it became up to 60 mV negative with respect to an electrode in the external solution. The *resting potential* across the membrane in the intact axon was thus about –60 mV, inside relative to outside. On stimulation of the axon by applying a shock at the far end, the amplitude of the *action potential* (Figure 2.3) – or *spike*, as it is often called – was found to be over 100 mV, so that at its peak the membrane potential was reversed by at least 40 mV. Typical values for isolated axons recorded with this type of electrode (Figure 2.4*a*) would be a resting potential of –60 mV and a spike of 110 mV, that is to say an internal potential of +50 mV at the peak of the spike. Records made with 0.5 µm electrodes for undissected axons *in situ* in the squid's mantle give slightly larger potentials, and the underswing or *positive phase* at the tail of the spike is no longer seen (Figure 2.4*b*). At 20 °C the duration of the spike is about 0.5 ms; the records in Figure 2.4 were made at a lower temperature.

As may be seen in Figure 2.4*c–h*, every kind of excitable tissue, from mammalian motor nerve to muscle and electric organ, gives a similar picture as far as the sizes of the resting and action potentials are concerned. The resting potential always lies between –60 and –95 mV, and the potential at the peak of the spike between +20 and +50 mV. However, the shapes and durations of the action potentials show considerable variation, their length ranging from 0.5 ms in a mammalian myelinated fibre to 0.5 s in a cardiac muscle fibre, with its characteristically prolonged plateau. But it is important to note that for a given fibre the shape and size of the action potential remain exactly the same as long as external conditions such as the temperature and the composition of the bathing solution are kept constant. As will be explained later, this is an essential consequence of the *all-or-nothing* behaviour of the propagated impulse.

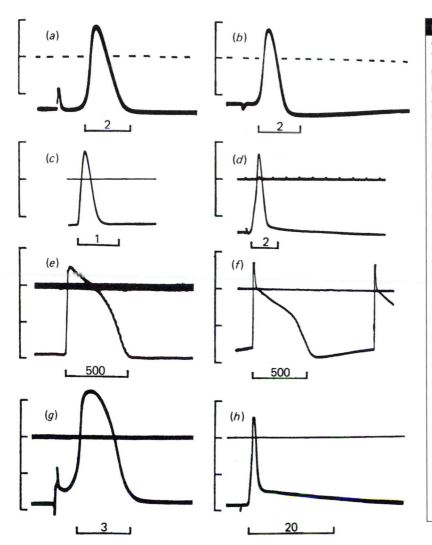

Figure 2.4 Intracellular records of resting and action potentials. The horizontal lines (dashed in (a) and (b)) indicate zero potential; positive potential upwards. Marks on the voltage scales are 50 mV apart. The number against each time scale is its length (ms). In some cases the action potential is preceded by a stimulus artifact: (a) squid axon *in situ* at 8.5 °C, recorded with 0.5 μm microelectrode; (b) squid axon isolated by dissection, at 12.5 °C, recorded with 100 μm longitudinal microelectrode; (c) myelinated fibre from dorsal root of cat; (d) cell body of motoneuron in spinal cord of cat; (e) muscle fibre in frog's heart; (f) Purkinje fibre in sheep's heart; (g) electroplate in electric organ of *Electrophorus electricus*; (h), isolated fibre from frog's sartorius muscle. ((a) and (b) recorded by A. L. Hodgkin and R. D. Keynes, from Hodgkin, 1958; (c) recorded by K. Krnjević; (d) from Brock, Coombs and Eccles, 1952; (e) recorded by B. F. Hoffman; (f) recorded by S. Weidmann, from Weidmann, 1956; (g) from Keynes and Martins-Ferreira, 1953; (h) from Hodgkin and Horowicz, 1957.)

2.3 | Extracellular recording of the nervous impulse

There are many experimental situations where it is impracticable to use intracellular electrodes, so that the passage of impulses can only be studied with the aid of external electrodes. It is therefore necessary to consider how the picture obtained with such electrodes is related to the potential changes at membrane level.

Since during the impulse the potential across the active membrane is reversed, making the outside negative with respect to the inside, the active region of the nerve becomes electrically negative relative to the resting region. With two electrodes placed far apart on an intact nerve, as in Figure 2.5a, an impulse set up by stimulation

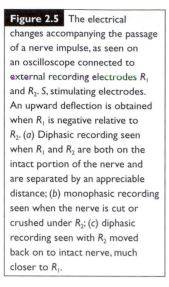

Figure 2.5 The electrical changes accompanying the passage of a nerve impulse, as seen on an oscilloscope connected to external recording electrodes R_1 and R_2. S, stimulating electrodes. An upward deflection is obtained when R_1 is negative relative to R_2. (*a*) Diphasic recording seen when R_1 and R_2 are both on the intact portion of the nerve and are separated by an appreciable distance; (*b*) monophasic recording seen when the nerve is cut or crushed under R_2; (*c*) diphasic recording seen with R_2 moved back on to intact nerve, much closer to R_1.

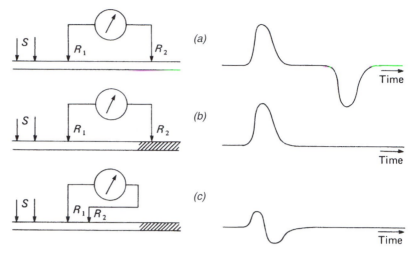

at the left-hand end first reaches R_1 and makes it temporarily negative, then traverses the stretch between R_1 and R_2, and finally arrives under R_2, where it gives rise to a mirror-image deflection on the oscilloscope. The resulting record is a *diphasic* one. If the nerve is cut or crushed under R2, the impulse is extinguished when it reaches this point, and the record becomes *monophasic* (Figure 2.5*b*). However, it is sometimes difficult to obtain the classical diphasic action potential of Figure 2.5*a* because the electrodes cannot be separated by a great enough distance. In a frog nerve at room temperature, the duration of the action potential is of the order of 1.5 ms, and the conduction velocity is about 20 m/s. The active region therefore occupies 30 mm, and altogether some 50 mm of nerve must be dissected, requiring a rather large frog, to give room for complete separation of the upward and downward deflections. When the electrodes are closer together than the length of the active region, there is a partial overlap between the phases, and the diphasic recording has a reduced amplitude and no central flat portion (Figure 2.5*c*).

A whole nerve trunk contains a mixture of fibres having widely different diameters, spike durations and conduction velocities, so that even a monophasic spike recording may have a complicated appearance. When a frog's sciatic nerve is stimulated strongly enough to excite all the fibres, an electrode placed near the point of stimulation will give a monophasic action potential that appears as a single wave, but a recording made at a greater distance will reveal several waves because of dispersion of the conducted spikes with distance. The three main groups of spikes are conventionally labelled A, B and C, and A may be subdivided into α, β and γ. In the experiment shown in Figure 2.6, for which a large American bullfrog was used at room temperature, the distance from the stimulating to the recording electrode was 131 mm. If the time for the foot of the wave to reach the recording electrode is read off the logarithmic scale of Figure 2.6*a*, it can be calculated that the rate of conduction was

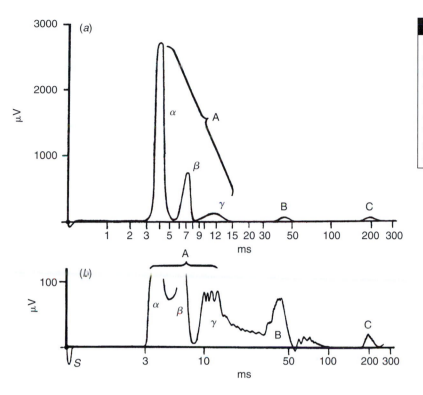

Figure 2.6 A monophasic recording of the compound action potential of a bullfrog's peroneal nerve at a conduction distance of 13.1 cm. Time shown in milliseconds on a logarithmic scale. Amplification for (b) is 10 times that for (a). S, stimulus artifact at zero time. (Redrawn after Erlanger and Gasser, 1937.)

41 mm/ms for α, 22 for β, 14 for γ, 4 for B and 0.7 for C. The conduction velocities in mammalian nerves are somewhat greater (100 for α, 60 for β, 40 for γ, 10 for B and 2 for C), partly because of the higher body temperature and partly because the fibres are larger.

This wide distribution of conduction velocities results from an equally wide variation in fibre diameter. A large nerve fibre conducts impulses faster than a small one. Several other characteristics of nerve fibres depend markedly on their size. Thus the smaller fibres need stronger shocks to excite them, so that the form of the volley recorded from a mixed nerve trunk is affected by the strength of the stimulus. With a weak shock, only the α wave appears; if the shock is stronger, then both α and β waves are seen, and so on. The amplitude of the voltage change picked up by an external recording electrode also varies with fibre diameter. On theoretical grounds it might be expected to vary with the square of diameter, but Gasser's reconstructions provide some support for the view that in practice the relationship is more nearly a linear one. In either case, the consequence is that when the electrical activity in a sensory nerve is recorded *in situ*, the picture is dominated by what is happening in the largest fibres, and it is difficult to see anything at all of the action potentials in the small nonmyelinated fibres.

While there is a wide range of fibre diameters in most nerve trunks, it is in most cases difficult to attribute particular functions to particular sizes of fibres. The sensory root of the spinal cord contains fibres giving A (that is α, β and γ) and C waves; the motor root yields α, γ and B waves, the latter going into the white ramus. It is generally believed that B fibres occur only in the preganglionic autonomic nerves, so that what is labelled B in Figure 2.6 might be better classified as subdivision δ of group A. The grey ramus, containing fibres belonging to the sympathetic system, shows mainly C waves. The fastest fibres (α) are either motor fibres activating voluntary muscles or afferent fibres conveying impulses from sensory receptors in these muscles. The γ motor fibres in mammals are connected to intrafusal muscle fibres in the muscle spindles, but in amphibia they innervate 'slow' as opposed to 'twitch' muscles (see Section 11.2). At least some of the fibres of the non-myelinated C group convey pain impulses, but they mainly belong to post-ganglionic autonomic nerves. The myelinated sensory fibres in peripheral nerves have also been classified according to their diameters into group I (20 to 12 μm), group II (12 to 4 μm) and group III (less than 4 μm). Functionally, the group I fibres are found only in nerves from muscles, subdivision IA being connected with annulo-spiral endings of muscle spindles, and the more slowly conducting IB fibres carrying impulses from Golgi tendon organs. The still slower fibres of groups II and III transmit other modes of sensation in both muscle and skin nerves.

2.4 | Excitation

Before considering the ionic basis of the mechanism of conduction of the nervous impulse, it is best to describe some facts concerning the process of excitation, that is to say the way in which the impulse is set up in nerve and muscle fibres. This order of treatment is, historically, that in which research on the subject developed, because progress towards a proper understanding of the details of the conduction mechanism was inevitably slow before the introduction of intracellular recording techniques, whereas excitation could be investigated with comparatively simple methods such as observing whether or not a muscle was induced to twitch.

A nerve can be stimulated by the local application of a number of agents that include electric current, pressure, heat, solutions containing substances like KCl, or optical excitation of genetically introduced photosensitive molecules such as channelrhodopsin-2 (Zhang *et al.*, 2006). However, it is most easily and conveniently stimulated by applying electric shocks. The most effective electric current is one which flows outwards across the membrane and so *depolarizes* it, that is to say reduces the size of the resting potential. The other agents listed above also act by causing a depolarization, pressure and heat doing so by damaging the membrane. A flow of current in the appropriate direction may be brought about either

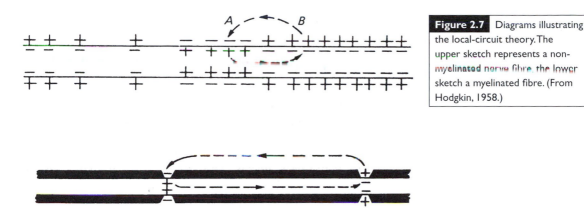

Figure 2.7 Diagrams illustrating the local-circuit theory. The upper sketch represents a non-myelinated nerve fibre, the lower sketch a myelinated fibre. (From Hodgkin, 1958.)

by applying a negative voltage pulse to a nearby electrode, making it *cathodal,* or through *local-circuit* action when an impulse set up further along the fibre reaches the stretch of membrane under consideration. It was suggested long ago that propagation of an impulse depends essentially on the flow of current in local circuits ahead of the active region which depolarizes the resting membrane, and causes it in turn to become active. The local-circuit theory is illustrated in Figure 2.7, which shows how current flowing from region *A* to region *B* in a non-myelinated fibre (upper diagram) results in movement of the active region towards the right. There are important differences that will be discussed later (see Chapter 6) between the current pathways in non-myelinated nerves or in muscle fibres on the one hand, and in myelinated fibres on the other (lower diagram), but the basic principle is the same in each case. The role of local circuits in the conduction of impulses has been accepted for some time, and is mentioned at this point in order to emphasize that in studying the effect of applied electric currents we are not concerned with a non-physiological and purely artificial way of setting up a nervous impulse, but are examining a process which forms an integral part of the normal mechanism of propagation.

The first concept that must be understood is that of a *threshold* stimulus. The smallest voltage which gives rise to a just-perceptible muscle twitch is the minimal or threshold stimulus. It is the voltage which is just large enough to stimulate one of the nerve fibres, and hence to cause contraction of the muscle fibres to which it is connected. If the nerve consisted only of a single fibre, it would be found that a further increase in the applied voltage would not make the twitch any stronger. This is because conduction is an *all-or-nothing* phenomenon: the stimulus either (if it is subthreshold) fails to set up an impulse, or (if it is threshold or above) sets up a full-sized impulse. No response of an intermediate size can be obtained by varying the stimulus strength, though of course the response may change if certain external conditions, for example temperature or ionic environment, are altered. In a multi-fibre preparation like the sciatic nerve there are hundreds of fibres whose thresholds are spread over quite

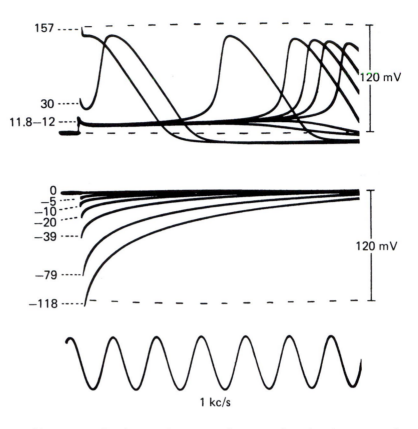

Figure 2.8 Threshold behaviour of the membrane potential in a squid giant axon at 6 °C. Shocks, whose strengths in nC/cm² membrane are shown against each trace, were applied to an internal wire electrode with a bare portion 15 mm long. The internal potential was recorded between a second wire 7 mm long opposite the centre of the stimulating wire and an electrode in the sea water outside. Depolarization is shown upwards. Sinusoidal wave at 1 kHz (1 kc/s) at bottom gives indication of timescale. (From Hodgkin *et al.*, 1952.)

a wide range of voltages. Hence an increase in stimulus strength above that which just excites the fibre with the lowest threshold results in excitation of more and more fibres, with a corresponding increase in the size of the muscle twitch. When the point is reached where the twitch ceases to increase any further, it can be taken that all the fibres in the nerve trunk are being triggered. This requires a *maximal* stimulus. A still larger (supra-maximal) shock does not produce a larger twitch.

A good example of the threshold behaviour of a single nerve fibre is provided by the experiment shown in Figure 2.8. Here an isolated squid giant axon was being stimulated over a length of 15 mm by applying brief shocks between a wire inserted axially into it and an external electrode, while the membrane potential was recorded internally by a second wire with a bare portion opposite the central 7 mm of the axon. The threshold for excitation was found to occur when a depolarizing shock of 11.8–12 nC/cm² membrane was applied to the stimulating wire. At this shock strength, the response arose after a delay of several milliseconds during which the membrane was depolarized by about 10 mV and was in a metastable condition, sometimes giving a spike and sometimes reverting to its resting state without generating one. When a larger shock was applied, the waiting period was reduced, but the size of the spike did not change appreciably. The lower part of the figure shows that when the direction of the shock was reversed to give inward

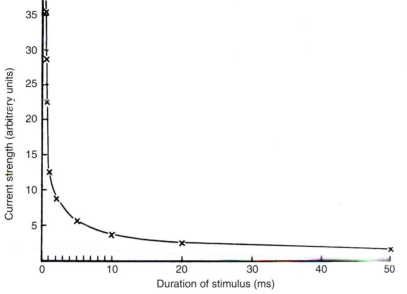

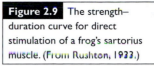

Figure 2.9 The strength–duration curve for direct stimulation of a frog's sartorius muscle. (From Rushton, 1933.)

current which polarized the membrane beyond the resting level, the displacement of the potential then decayed exponentially back to the resting value. The changes in the ionic permeability of the membrane that are responsible for this behaviour are explained in Chapter 3.

An important variable in investigating the excitability of a nerve is the duration of the shock. In measurements of the threshold, it is found that for long shocks the applied current reaches an irreducible minimum known as the *rheobase*. When the duration is reduced, a stronger shock is necessary to reach the threshold, so that the *strength–duration curve* relating shock strength to shock duration takes the form shown in Figure 2.9. The essential requirement for eliciting the action potential is that the membrane should be depolarized to a critical level whose existence is shown clearly by Figure 2.8. When the shock duration is reduced, more current must flow outwards if the membrane potential is to attain this critical level before the end of the shock. It follows that for short shocks a roughly constant total quantity of electricity has to be applied, and in Figure 2.8 the shock strength was therefore expressed in nC/cm² membrane.

For a short period after the passage of an impulse, the threshold for stimulation is raised, so that if a nerve is stimulated twice in quick succession, it may not respond to the second stimulus. The *absolute refractory period* is the brief interval after a successful stimulus when no second shock, however large, can elicit another spike. Its duration is roughly equal to that of the spike, which in mammalian A fibres at body temperature is of the order of 0.4 ms, or in frog nerve at 15 °C is about 2 ms. It is followed by the *relative refractory period*, during which a second response can be obtained if a strong enough shock is applied. This in turn is sometimes succeeded

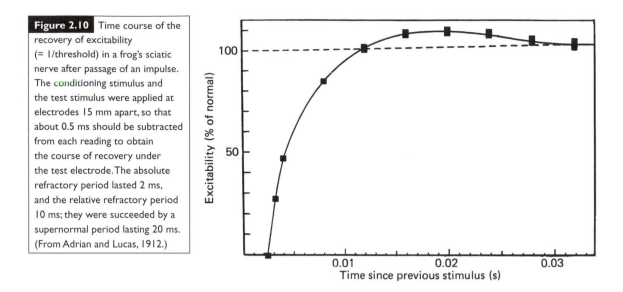

Figure 2.10 Time course of the recovery of excitability (= 1/threshold) in a frog's sciatic nerve after passage of an impulse. The conditioning stimulus and the test stimulus were applied at electrodes 15 mm apart, so that about 0.5 ms should be subtracted from each reading to obtain the course of recovery under the test electrode. The absolute refractory period lasted 2 ms, and the relative refractory period 10 ms; they were succeeded by a supernormal period lasting 20 ms. (From Adrian and Lucas, 1912.)

by a phase of supernormality when the excitability may be slightly greater than normal. Figure 2.10 illustrates the time course of the changes in excitability (= 1/threshold) in a frog sciatic nerve after the passage of an action potential.

The refractoriness of a nerve after conducting an impulse sets an upper limit to spike frequency. During the relative refractory period, both the spike size and the conduction velocity are subnormal, as well as the excitability, so that two impulses traversing a long length of nerve must be separated by a minimum interval if the second one is to be full-sized. A mammalian A fibre can conduct up to 1000 impulses/s, but the spikes would be small and would decline further during sustained stimulation. In A fibres, recovery is complete after about 3 ms, so that the frequency limit for full-sized spikes is 300/s. Even this repetition rate is not often attained in the living animal, though certain sensory nerves may exceed it occasionally for short bursts of impulses.

3

The ionic permeability of the nerve membrane

3.1 | Structure of the cell membrane

All living cells are surrounded by a plasma membrane composed of lipids and proteins, whose main function is to control the passage of substances into and out of the cell. In general, the role of the lipids is to furnish a continuous matrix that is impermeable even to the smallest ions, in which proteins are embedded to provide selective pathways for the transport of ions and organic molecules both down and against the prevailing gradients of chemical activity. The ease with which a molecule can cross a cell membrane depends to some extent on its size, but more importantly on its charge and lipid solubility. Hence the lipid matrix can exclude completely all large water-soluble molecules and also small charged molecules and ions, but is permeable to water and small uncharged molecules like urea. The nature of the transport pathways is dependent on the specific function of the cell under consideration. In the case of nerve and muscle, the pathways that are functionally important in connection with the conduction mechanism are: (1) the voltage-sensitive sodium and potassium channels peculiar to electrically excitable membranes, (2) the ligand-gated channels at synapses that transfer excitation onwards from the nerve terminal, and (3) the ubiquitous sodium pump, which is responsible in all types of cell for the extrusion of sodium ions from the interior.

The essential feature of membrane lipids that enables them to provide a structure with electrically insulating properties, i.e. to act as a barrier to the free passage of ions, is their possession of hydrophilic (polar) head groups and hydrophobic (non-polar) tails. When lipids are spread on the surface of water, they form a stable monolayer in which the polar ends are in contact with the water and the non-polar hydrocarbon chains are oriented more or less at right angles to the plane of the surface. The cell membrane consists basically of two lipid monolayers arranged back-to-back with the polar head groups facing outwards, so that the resulting sandwich interposes between the aqueous phases on either side of an

Figure 3.1 Schematic diagram of the structure of a cell membrane. Two layers of phospholipid molecules face one another with their fatty-acid chains forming a continuous hydrocarbon layer (*HC*) and their polar head groups (*Pol*) in the aqueous phase. The selective pathways for ion transport are provided by proteins extending across the membrane, which have a central hydrophobic section with non-polar side chains (*NP*) and hydrophilic portions projecting on either side.

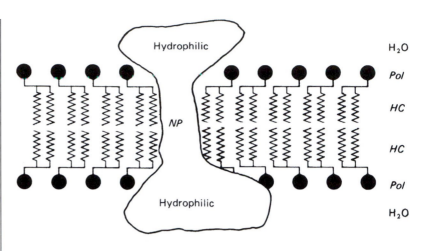

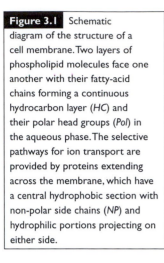

Cholesterol

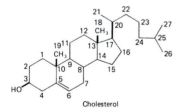

Phosphatidylcholine (lecithin)

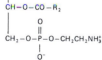

Phosphatidylethanolamine (cephalin)

Figure 3.2 The chemical structure of cholesterol and two neutral phospholipids.

uninterrupted hydrocarbon phase whose thickness is roughly twice the hydrocarbon chain length (Figure 3.1). Lipid *bilayers* of this type can readily be prepared artificially, and such so-called 'black membranes' have provided a valuable model for the study of some of the properties of real cell membranes. The chemical structure of the phospholipids of which cell membranes are mainly composed is shown in Figure 3.2. They have a glycerol backbone esterified to two fatty acids and phosphoric acid, forming a phosphatidic acid with which alcohols like choline or ethanolamine are combined through another ester linkage to give the neutral phospholipids lecithin and cephalin, or an amino acid like serine is linked to give negatively charged phosphatidylserine. Another constituent of cell membranes is cholesterol, whose physical properties are similar to those of a lipid because of the −OH group attached to C-3. Spin-label and deuterium nuclear magnetic resonance studies of lipid bilayers have shown that the hydrocarbon chains are packed rather loosely so that the interior of the bilayer behaves like a liquid. With a chain length of 18 carbon atoms, the effective thickness of the hydrophobic region is about 3.0 nm, which is consistent with the observed electrical capacitance of 1 $\mu F/cm^2$ membrane and a dielectric constant of 3.

Thanks to the advent of cDNA sequencing studies (see Section 5.1), our understanding of the organization of the protein moiety of the membrane has made rapid advances in recent years. Sections stained with permanganate or osmic acid for high-resolution electron microscopy (Figure 3.3) show the membrane in all types of cell to appear as two uniform lines separated by a space, the width of the whole structure being about 7.5 nm. This fits with the model proposed by Davson and Danielli (1943), according to which the lipid bilayer is stabilized by a thin coating of protein molecules on either side, and the electron-dense stain is taken up by the polar groups of the phospholipids and of the proteins associated with them. However, an examination of freeze-fractured membranes under

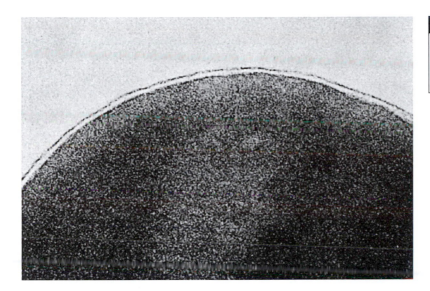

Figure 3.3 Electron micrograph at high magnification of the cell membrane stained with osmic acid. (Reproduced by courtesy of Professor J. D. Robertson.)

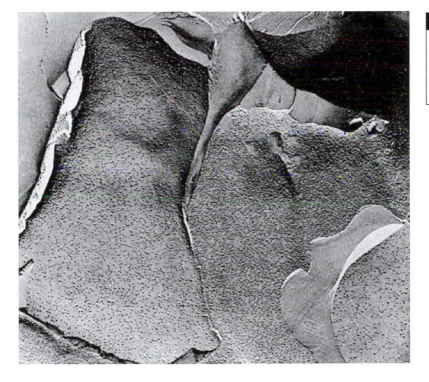

Figure 3.4 Electron micrograph of a freeze-fracture preparation of a cell membrane. The proteins appear as globular indentations. (Reproduced by courtesy of Professor J. D. Robertson.)

the electron microscope (Figure 3.4) indicates that those proteins which traverse the bilayer to form specific ion-conducting or ion-pumping pathways are sometimes visible as globular indentations or projections. Such membrane proteins have a central non-polar section that is at home in the hydrophobic environment provided by the hydrocarbon chains of the lipids, together with polar and often

Table 3.1	*Ionic concentrations in frog muscle fibres and plasma*	
	Concentration in fibre water (mM)	Concentration in plasma water (mM)
K^+	124	2.3
Na^+	3.6	108.8
Ca^{2+}	4.9	2.1
Mg^{2+}	14.0	1.3
Cl^-	1.5	77.9
HCO_3^-	12.4	26.6
Phosphocreatine	35.2	–
Organic anions	c. 45	c. 14

Notes: These figures are calculated from values given by Conway (1957). At pH 7.0, phosphocreatine carries two negative charges; the remaining deficit in intracellular anions is made up by proteins. Approximate values are denoted c.

glycosidic portions extending into the aqueous medium both inside and outside. Whether they are held in a fixed position in the membrane by internal fibrils, or are free to rotate and move laterally, is not always clear, but it may well be that some freedom of movement is necessary for their normal functioning.

3.2 | Distribution of ions in nerve and muscle

With the advent of flame photometry and other microanalytical techniques there is no difficulty in determining the quantities of ions present in a small sample of tissue. In order to arrive at the true intracellular concentrations, it is necessary to make corrections for the contents of the extracellular space, which may be done after measuring its size with the aid of a substance like inulin to which the cell membrane is impermeable. Table 3.1 gives a simplified balance sheet of the ionic concentrations in frog muscle fibres and blood plasma determined in this way.

In the case of the squid giant axon it is possible to extrude the axoplasm, just as toothpaste is squeezed from a tube, and so to obtain samples uncontaminated by extracellular ions. Table 3.2 shows the resulting ionic balance sheet.

The main features of the distribution of ions which all excitable tissues have in common are that the intracellular K^+ is 20 to 50 times higher in the cytoplasm than in the blood, and that for Na^+ and Cl^- the situation is reversed. The total amount of ions is, of course, about four times greater in a marine invertebrate like the squid, whose blood is isotonic with sea water, than it is in an amphibian like the frog, which lives in fresh water, but the concentration ratios are not very different. The principal anion in the external medium

Table 3.2	Ionic concentrations in squid axoplasm and blood	
	Concentration in axoplasm (mM)	Concentration in blood (mM)
K⁺	400	20
Na⁺	50	440
Ca²⁺	0.4	10
Mg²⁺	10	54
Cl⁻	123	560
Arginine phosphate	5	–
Isethionate	250	–
Other organic anions	c. 110	c. 30

These values are taken from Hodgkin (1958) and Keynes (1963). Approximate values are denoted c.

is chloride, but inside the cells its place is taken by a variety of non-penetrating organic anions. The problem of achieving a balance between intracellular anions and cations is most severe in marine invertebrates, and is met by the presence either of large amounts of aspartate and glutamate or, in squid, of isethionate.

3.3 | The genesis of the resting potential

When a membrane selectively permeable to a given ion separates two solutions containing different concentrations of that ion, an electrical potential difference is set up across it. In order to understand how this comes about, consider a compartment within which the ionic concentrations are $[K]_i$ and $[Cl]_i$, and outside which they are $[K]_o$ and $[Cl]_o$, bounded by a membrane that can discriminate perfectly between K^+ and Cl^- ions, allowing K^+ to pass freely, but being totally impermeable to Cl^-. If $[K]_i$ is greater than $[K]_o$ there will initially be a net outward movement of K^+ down the concentration gradient, but each K^+ ion escaping from the compartment unaccompanied by a Cl^- ion will tend to make the outside of the membrane electrically positive. The direction of the electric field set up by this separation of charge will be such as to assist the entry of K^+ ions into the compartment and hinder their exit. A state of equilibrium will quickly be reached in which the opposed influences of the concentration and electrical gradients on the ionic movements will exactly balance one another, and although there will be a continuous flux of ions crossing the membrane in each direction, there will be no further net movement.

The argument may be placed on a quantitative basis by equating the chemical work involved in the transfer of K^+ from one concentration to the other with the electrical work involved in the transfer against the potential gradient. In order to move 1 gram-mole of the univalent K^+ from inside to outside, the chemical work that has to be done is $RT \log_e\{[K]_o/[K]_i\}$. The corresponding electrical work is $-EF$, where E is the membrane potential, inside relative to outside, and F is the charge carried by 1 gram-equivalent of ions. At equilibrium, no net work is done, and the sum of the two is zero, whence

$$E = (RT/F) \log_e\{[K]_o/[K]_i\} \tag{3.1}$$

This relationship was first derived by the German physical chemist Nernst in the nineteenth century, and the equilibrium potential E_K for a membrane permeable exclusively to K^+ ions is known as the *Nernst potential* for K^+. The values of R and F are such that at room temperature the potential is given by

$$E_K = 25 \log_e\{[K]_o/[K]_i\}\ mV = 58 \log_{10}\{[K]_o/[K]_i\}\ mV \tag{3.2}$$

An e-fold change in concentration ratio therefore corresponds to a 25 mV change in potential, or a tenfold change to 58 mV.

On examining the applicability of the Nernst relation to the situation in nerve and muscle, it is found (Figure 3.5) that it is well obeyed at high external K^+ concentrations, but that for small values of $[K]_o$ the potential alters less steeply than Equation (3.2) predicts. It is evident that the membrane does not in fact maintain a perfect selectivity for K^+ over the whole concentration range, and that the effect of the other ions which are present must be considered. In order to derive a theoretical expression relating the membrane potential to the permeabilities and concentrations of all the ions in the system, whether positively or negatively charged, some assumption has to

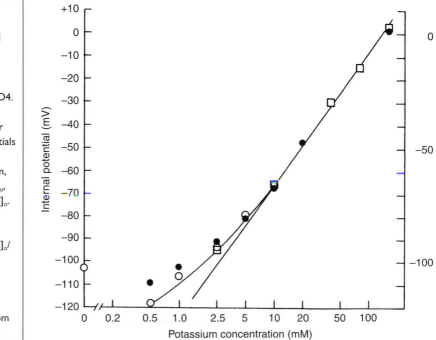

Figure 3.5 Variation in the resting potential of frog muscle fibres with the external K^+ concentration $[K]_o$. The measurements were made in a chloride-free sulfate-Ringer's solution containing 8 mM-CaSO4. Square symbols are potentials measured after equilibrating for 10 to 60 min; circles are potentials measured 20 to 60 s after a sudden change in concentration, filled ones after increase in $[K]_o$, open ones after decrease in $[K]_o$. For large $[K]_o$s the measured potentials agree well with the Nernst equation, $V = 58 \log\{[K]_o/[K]_i\}$, taking $[K]i$ as 140 mM. The deviation at low $[K]_o$ can partly be explained by taking $P_{Na}/P_K = 0.01$, so that $V = 58 \log\{\{[K]_o - 0.01[Na]_o\}/140\}$. (From Hodgkin and Horowicz, 1959.)

be made as to the manner in which the electric field varies within the membrane. Such an expression was first produced by Goldman, who showed that if the field was the same at all points across the membrane, the potential was given by

$$E = (RT/F)\log_e\{\{P_K[K]_o+P_{Na}[Na]_o+P_{Cl}[Cl]_i\}/\{P_K[K]_i+P_{Na}[Na]_i+P_{Cl}[Cl]_o\}\} \quad (3.3)$$

where the Ps are permeability coefficients for the various ions, and the suffixes o and i indicate external and internal concentrations respectively. Although the *constant field equation* has been shown in practice to fit rather well with experimental observation over a wide range of conditions, it does not follow that the field is indeed truly constant. Equation (3.3) is, nevertheless, empirically very valuable for describing the behaviour of a membrane permeable to more than one species of ion. Thus in the experiment of Figure 3.5, the deviation of the measured potential from a line with a slope of 58 mV can be accounted for nicely by taking P_{Na} to be 100 times smaller than P_K.

3.4 | The Donnan equilibrium system in muscle

Cells have an unequal but stable transmembrane distribution of ions. An important advance towards an understanding of these ionic inequalities was made in 1941 when Boyle and Conway pointed out that the type of equilibrium for diffusible and non-diffusible ions characterized by Donnan might apply in muscle cells. In a Donnan system consisting of two compartments separated by a membrane, there are no net ion fluxes because the equilibrium potential for each diffusible ion is equal to the membrane potential. The transmembrane concentration ratios of each monovalent ion must therefore be equal, since the same membrane potential is common to all of them. Boyle and Conway (1941) showed experimentally that in frog sartorius muscle the relationship

$$\{[K]_o/[K]_i\}=\{[Cl]_i/[Cl]_o\} \quad (3.4)$$

was duly obeyed, the ratio for K^+ ions being the inverse of that for Cl^- ions because of their opposite charges. Subsequent observations by Hodgkin and Horowicz on the effect of sudden changes in $[Cl]_o$ on the membrane potential of frog muscle fibres have borne out their conclusions in every respect.

As shown by Equations (3.2) and (3.3), the magnitude of the K^+ concentration gradient is an important determinant of the magnitude of the membrane potential. However, this requires low intracellular $[Cl^-]$ (Equation 3.4). Thus, a further requirement for the operation of a Donnan equilibrium is the presence of sufficient non-diffusible intracellular anions, as well as sufficient non-diffusible extracellular cations to achieve both an electrical balance between the anions and cations in each compartment, and an osmotic balance between the total solutes on the two sides. Boyle and Conway's proposition that K+ and Cl- can be regarded as diffusible ions and Na+ as non-diffusible went an appreciable way towards explaining the observed facts. More recent work (Fraser and Huang, 2004; Fraser *et al.*, 2005; Usher-Smith *et al.*, 2009) has shown that the magnitude of the fixed negative charge then determines the maximum K+ concentration gradient.

3.5 | The active transport of ions

The Donnan equilibrium hypothesis required that the muscle membrane should be completely impermeable to Na+. When the radioactive isotope ^{24}Na became available, this was soon found not to be so, for about half of the intracellular sodium in the fibres of a frog's sartorius muscle turned out to be exchanged with the sodium in the external medium in the course of one hour. Moreover, experiments on giant axons from squid and cuttlefish showed that after dissection there was a steady gain of sodium and loss of potassium that if not counteracted would eventually have led to an equalization of the sodium and potassium contents of the axoplasm. It became clear that in actuality the resting cell membrane does have a finite permeability to Na+ ions, but that the inward leakage of sodium is offset by the operation of a *sodium pump*, which extrudes sodium at a rate which ensures that in the living animal [Na]$_i$ is kept roughly constant. As far as sodium and potassium are concerned, the resulting situation should be described as a steady state rather than an equilibrium, though for experiments like those carried out by Boyle and Conway the effect is the same. Since the expulsion of Na+ ions from the cell takes place against both an electrical gradient and a concentration gradient, it involves the performance of electrochemical work and requires a supply of energy from cell metabolism. The process is therefore termed *active transport*.

Giant axons have provided particularly favourable experimental material for radioactive tracer studies on the mechanism of the sodium pump. Figure 3.6 shows the results of an experiment in which the sodium efflux from a *Sepia* axon loaded with ^{24}Na and bathed in a non-radioactive medium was measured by counting samples of the bathing solution collected at 10 min intervals. The resting efflux was found to be roughly constant when calculated in moles of sodium per unit area of membrane per unit time, its average value at room temperature being around 40 pmole/cm^2 s. The linear decline seen in Figures 3.6 and 3.7 when the actual counts are plotted arises from the gradual dilution of the internal radioactivity by inactive sodium entering the axon as the experiment proceeds. When, however, the metabolic inhibitor 2,4-dinitrophenol (DNP) was added to the external medium, the counting rate fell quickly to about one-thirtieth of its previous level. The effect was reversible, and on washing away the DNP the efflux soon recovered. Axons treated with cyanide or azide behaved in a similar fashion. Since

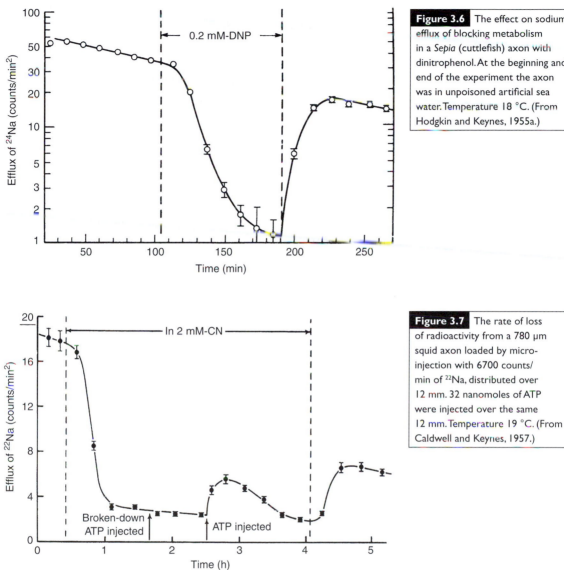

Figure 3.6 The effect on sodium efflux of blocking metabolism in a *Sepia* (cuttlefish) axon with dinitrophenol. At the beginning and end of the experiment the axon was in unpoisoned artificial sea water. Temperature 18 °C. (From Hodgkin and Keynes, 1955a.)

Figure 3.7 The rate of loss of radioactivity from a 780 µm squid axon loaded by micro-injection with 6700 counts/min of ^{22}Na, distributed over 12 mm. 32 nanomoles of ATP were injected over the same 12 mm. Temperature 19 °C. (From Caldwell and Keynes, 1957.)

all these inhibitors are known to act by blocking the production of the energy-rich compound adenosine triphosphate (ATP) by oxidative phosphorylation in the mitochondria, the implication was that the sodium pump was driven by energy derived from the terminal phosphate bond of ATP.

The role of ATP as the immediate source of energy for sodium extrusion was further examined by testing its ability to restore the sodium efflux when injected into cyanide-poisoned axons. Figure 3.7 shows that ATP injection did bring about some degree of recovery of the efflux, but it turned out that a complete recovery was only obtained if the ratio of [ATP] to [ADP] in the axoplasm was made reasonably large. This could be achieved by the injection of arginine

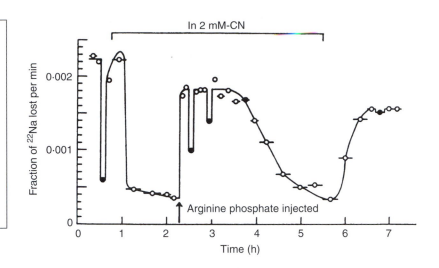

Figure 3.8 The effect on the efflux of labelled sodium from a squid giant axon of first blocking metabolism with cyanide and then injecting a large quantity of arginine phosphate. Open circles show efflux with $[K]_o = 10$ mM; filled circles show efflux into a potassium-free solution. Immediately after the injection the mean internal concentration of arginine phosphate was 33 mM. Temperature 18 °C. (From Caldwell *et al.*, 1960.)

phosphate, which serves as a reservoir for high-energy phosphate in the tissues of invertebrates through the reaction:

ADP + arginine phosphate $\rightarrow$ ATP + arginine.

An important characteristic of the sodium pump is its dependence for normal working on the presence of potassium in the external medium. Thus when at the beginning of the experiment illustrated in Figure 3.8 $[K]_o$ was reduced to zero, the unpoisoned sodium efflux fell to about a quarter of its normal size. After the cyanide had taken effect, a large amount of arginine phosphate was injected into the axon. This duly brought the efflux back to normal, but only during the first hour was it sensitive to the removal of potassium. In a similar way, the efflux that reappeared on washing away the cyanide only regained its potassium sensitivity when sufficient time had been allowed for the ATP/ADP ratio to return to normal. The requirement of the sodium pump for external K^+ suggested that there might be an obligatory coupling between the extrusion of sodium and an uptake of K^+. Parallel measurements of the efflux of ^{24}Na and the influx of ^{42}K have shown that this is indeed the case, and that in many tissues the coupling ratio is normally 3:2, i.e. for every three Na^+ ions that leave the cell, two K^+ ions are taken up. If the coupling ratio were exactly 1:1, the sodium pump would be electrically neutral in the sense that it would bring about no net transfer of charge across the membrane. A coupling ratio greater than unity implies that the sodium pump is electrogenic, and causes a separation of charge which tends to hyperpolarize the membrane. The after-potential that succeeds the impulse in small non-myelinated nerve fibres is thought to arise in this way from an acceleration of the sodium pump, and the pumping of ions in many other situations has now been shown to be electrogenic to some degree.

The sodium pump occurs universally in the cells of higher animals, and can be identified with the enzyme system Na,K-ATPase, first extracted from crab nerve by Skou in Aarhus University (reviewed in: Skou, 1998), Research on the chemistry of Na,K-ATPase has depended heavily on the exploitation of the inhibitory action of glycosides like ouabain and digoxin, which in micromolar concentrations block both the active fluxes of sodium and potassium in intact tissues, and the splitting of ATP by purified enzyme preparations. By measuring the binding of ouabain labelled with tritium, it is possible to estimate the number of sodium pumping sites in a unit area of membrane, assuming that each site binds one molecule of ouabain. In the squid giant axon there are several thousand sites per square micrometre of membrane, while in the smallest non-myelinated fibres the density of sites is about a tenth as great.

Although the extrusion of Na^+ and intake of K^+ ions by the sodium pump is quickly halted by ouabain or any metabolic inhibitor which deprives the pump of its supply of ATP, neither treatment has any immediate effect on electrical excitability. Figure 3.9 shows the results of an experiment in which the sodium influx into a squid giant axon was measured by soaking it for a few minutes in a solution containing ^{24}Na and then mounting it above a Geiger counter in a stream of unlabelled artificial sea water. While sodium was being actively extruded from the axon, the counting rate fell steadily, but on the addition of DNP to the sea water bathing the axon, the counts remained constant. When the DNP was washed away, the sodium pump started up again. The rate of gain of radioactivity during the periods of exposure to ^{24}Na was increased by a factor of about 10 by stimulation at 50 shocks/s, but the extra entry of ^{24}Na was the

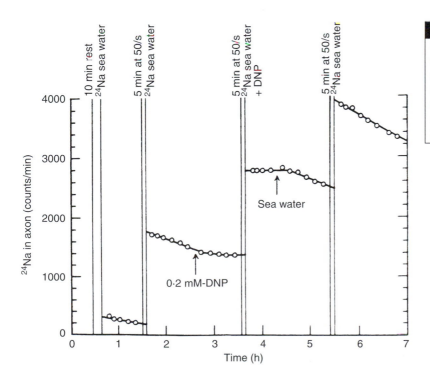

Figure 3.9 The lack of effect of dinitrophenol on the sodium entry during stimulation of a squid axon. The resting sodium influx for the first period of immersion in ^{24}Na sea water was 50 pmole/cm^2. Temperature 17 °C. (From Hodgkin and Keynes, 1955a.)

Table 3.3 | *Comparison of the properties of the sodium and potassium channels with those of the sodium pump*

	Sodium and potassium channels	Sodium pump
Direction of ion movements	Down the electrochemical gradient	Against the electrochemical gradient
Source of energy	Pre-existing electrochemical gradients	ATP
Voltage dependence	Regenerative link between potential and sodium conductance	Independent of potential
Blocking agents	Tetrodotoxin blocks Na^+ channels at 10^{-8} M Tetramethylammonium blocks K^+ channels Ouabain has no effect	Tetrodotoxin has no effect Tetramethylammonium has no effect at 10^{-3} M Ouabain blocks at 10^{-7} M
External Ca^{2+}	Increase in [Ca] raises threshold for excitation; decrease in [Ca] lowers threshold	No effect
Selectivity	Li^+ is not distinguished from Na^+	Li^+ is pumped much more slowly than Na^+
Effect of temperature	Rate of opening and closing of channels has large temperature coefficient, but maximum conductances have a small one	Velocity of pumping has a large temperature coefficient
Density of distribution in the membrane	Squid axon has 290 TTX-binding sites per μm^2 Rabbit vagus has 100 TTX-binding sites per μm^2	Squid axon has 4000 ouabain-binding sites per μm^2 Rabbit vagus has 750 ouabain-binding sites per μm^2
Maximum rate of movement of Na^+	100 000 pmol/cm^2 s during rising phase of action potential	60 pmole/cm^2 s of Na^+ at room temperature
Metabolic inhibitors	No effect; electrical activity is normal in axon perfused with pure salt solution	1 mM-cyanide or 0.2 mM-dinitrophenol block as soon as ATP is exhausted

same whether or not the sodium pump had been blocked. Washing out experiments showed that the accelerated outward movement of [24]Na during the impulse (see Sections 3.5 and 4.2) was affected equally little by DNP.

It follows from this evidence and many other considerations summarized in Table 3.3 that, as indicated diagrammatically in Figure 3.10, the pathways for the active and passive transport of ions across the membrane function quite independently of one another. This can be demonstrated most clearly in giant axons because of their large volume-to-surface ratio. Perhaps the most striking example of the independence of the pump and spike mechanisms was provided by Baker *et al.* when they showed that

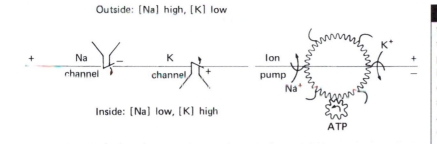

Outside: [Na] high, [K] low

Inside: [Na] low, [K] high

Figure 3.10 There are two types of ion channel traversing the nerve membrane. The sodium pump responsible for transporting ions uphill and so creating the concentration gradients is shown as a bucket system driven by ATP. The sodium and potassium channels involved in excitation are shown as funnel-shaped structures whose opening is controlled by the electric field across the membrane. In this diagram they are in the resting state with the charged gates held closed by the membrane potential. On depolarization of the membrane the gates open and permit ions to flow downhill.

a squid axon whose axoplasm had been extruded and replaced by a pure solution of potassium sulfate was nevertheless capable of conducting over 400 000 impulses before becoming exhausted. In a small non-myelinated nerve fibre the downhill ionic movements during the nervous impulse are much larger in relation to the reservoir of ions built up by the sodium pump, so that blockage of active transport does, after a relatively short while, affect the conduction mechanism indirectly by reducing the size of the ionic concentration gradients.

Membrane permeability changes during excitation

4.1 | The impedance change during the spike

An important landmark in the development of theories about the mechanism of conduction was the demonstration by Cole and Curtis in 1939 that the passage of an impulse in the squid giant axon was accompanied by a substantial drop in the electrical impedance of its membrane. The axon was mounted in a trough between two plate electrodes connected in one arm of a Wheatstone bridge circuit (Figure 4.1) for the measurement of resistance and capacitance in parallel. The output of the bridge was displayed on a cathode-ray oscilloscope, and R_v and C_v were adjusted to give a balance, and therefore zero output, with the axon at rest. When the axon was stimulated at one end, the bridge went briefly out of balance (Figure 4.2) with a time course very similar to that of the action potential. The change was shown to be due entirely to a reduction in the resistance of the membrane from a resting value of about 1000 Ω cm^2 to an active one in the neighbourhood of 25 Ω cm^2. The membrane capacitance of about 1 μF/cm^2 did not alter measurably.

4.2 | The sodium hypothesis

Cole and Curtis's results were not wholly unexpected, because it had long been supposed that there was some kind of collapse in the selectivity of the membrane towards K$^+$ ions during the impulse. However, a year or two later both they and Hodgkin and Huxley succeeded in recording internal potentials for the first time, and it became apparent that, as has been seen in Figure 2.4, the membrane potential did not just fall towards zero at the peak of the spike, but instead was reversed by quite a few millivolts. This unexpected overshoot could not possibly be accounted for by any hypothesis involving a reduction in the ionic selectivity of the nerve membrane, but required a radically different type of explanation.

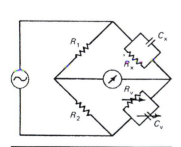

Figure 4.1 Wheatstone bridge circuit used for the measurement of resistance and capacitance in parallel.

(a)

(b)

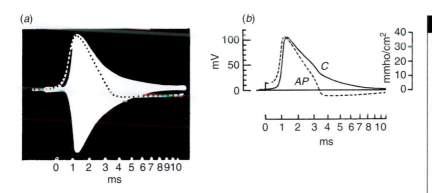

Figure 4.2 The time course of the impedance change during the conducted action potential in a squid giant axon recorded by Cole and Curtis (1939): (a) double exposure of the unbalance of the impedance bridge and of the monophasic action potential at one of the impedance electrodes; the time marks at the bottom are 1 ms apart; (b) superimposed plots of the membrane conductance increase (C) and of the action potential (AP) after correction for amplifier response.

None was forthcoming until in 1949 Hodgkin and Katz put forward the *sodium hypothesis of nervous conduction*. Noting that because the external sodium concentration $[Na]_o$ is greater than the internal concentration $[Na]_i$, the Nernst equilibrium potential for sodium (E_{Na}) is reversed in polarity compared with E_K, they suggested that excitation involves a rapid and highly specific increase in the permeability of the membrane to Na^+ ions, which shifts the membrane potential from its resting level near E_K to a new value that approaches E_{Na}. The first piece of evidence in support of this theory was the fact that nerves are indeed rendered inexcitable by Na^+-free solutions. As Overton showed long ago for frog muscle, only Li^+ ions can fully replace Na^+, though it is now known that there are several small organic cations like hydroxylamine which can act as partial Na^+ substitutes; and certain excitable tissues have a Ca^{2+}-dependent spike mechanism. As may be seen in Figure 4.3, replacement of part of the external Na^+ by glucose reduced both the rate of rise of the action potential and its height. The rate of rise was directly proportional to $[Na]_o$, while in accordance with Equations (3.2) and (3.3) the slope of the line relating spike height to $\log_{10}[Na]_o$ was close to 58 mV until the point was reached where conduction failed. Subsequent experiments have shown that a similar relation holds good when $[Na]_i$ is varied.

In order to change the potential across a membrane whose capacitance is 1 μF/cm^2, from −60 mV at rest to +50 mV at the peak of the spike, the total quantity of charge transferred must be 110 nC/cm^2, which would be carried by 1.1 picomoles of a monovalent ion crossing 1 cm^2 of membrane. A crucial test of the validity of the sodium hypothesis was therefore to measure the net entry of sodium into the fibre and the net loss of potassium from it during the passage of an impulse. Using the technique of radioactivation analysis, Keynes and Lewis (1951) found that in stimulated *Sepia* axons there was a net gain of 3.8 pmole Na/cm^2 impulse and a net loss of 3.6 pmole K/cm^2 impulse, while in squid axons the corresponding figures were 3.5 pmole Na and 3.0 pmole K. The measured ionic movements were thus more than large enough to comply with the theory. It was not surprising that they were actually somewhat greater than

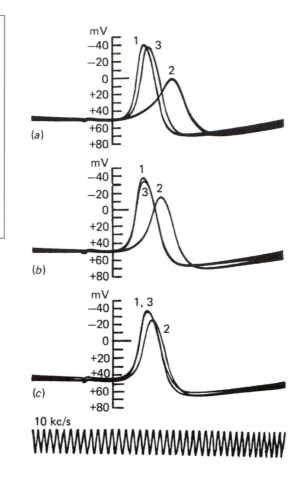

Figure 4.3 The effect of reducing the external Na⁺ concentration on the action potential in a squid giant axon. In each set of records, record 1 shows the response with the axon in sea water, record 2 in the experimental solution and record 3 in sea water again. The solutions were prepared by mixing sea water and an isotonic dextrose solution, the proportions of sea water being: (a), 33%; (b), 50%; (c), 71%. (From Hodgkin and Katz, 1949.)

the theoretical minimum, because it was reasonable to expect that there might be some exchange of potassium for sodium over the top of the spike in addition to the net uptake of sodium during its upstroke and the net loss of potassium during its falling phase. Experiments with ^{24}Na like that illustrated in Figure 4.4 showed that there was an analogous exchange of labelled sodium during the spike as well as a net entry, for the extra inward movement of radioactive sodium was estimated as 10 pmole/cm^2 impulse, and the extra outward movement as about 6 pmole/cm^2 impulse, the difference between the two figures being in good agreement with the analytical results.

The essential new property of the membrane envisaged by the sodium hypothesis was its possession of voltage-sensitive mechanisms providing appropriate control of its Na⁺ and K⁺ permeabilities. The sequence of events supposed to occur during the action potential may be summarized as follows: when the membrane is depolarized by an outward flow of current, caused either by an applied cathode or by the proximity of an active region where

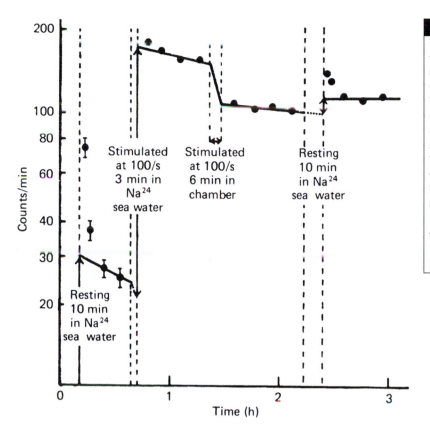

Figure 4.4 The movements of [24]Na in a stimulated *Sepia* axon whose diameter was 170 μm. The axon was alternately exposed to artificial sea water containing [24]Na, and mounted in a stream of inactive sea water above a Geiger counter for measurement of the amount of radioactivity taken up. The loss of counts during the first 10 min after exposure to [24]Na resulted from washing away extracellular Na⁺, and was ignored. For the entry of [24]Na, 1 count/min was equivalent to 42.5×10^{-12} mole Na/cm axon. Temperature 14 °C. (From Keynes, 1951.)

the membrane potential is already reversed, its Na⁺ permeability immediately rises, and there is a net inward movement of Na⁺ ions, flowing down the Na⁺ concentration gradient. If the initial depolarization opens the Na⁺ channels far enough, Na⁺ enters faster than K⁺ can leave, and this causes the membrane potential to drop still further. The extra depolarization increases the Na⁺ permeability even more, accelerating the change of membrane potential in a regenerative fashion. The linkage between Na⁺ permeability and membrane potential forms, as shown in Figure 4.5, is a *positive-feedback* mechanism. The entry of Na⁺ does not continue indefinitely, being halted partly because the membrane potential soon reaches a level close to E_{Na}, where the net inward driving force acting on Na⁺ ions becomes zero, and partly because the rise in Na⁺ permeability decays inexorably with time from the moment when it is first triggered, this process being termed *inactivation*. After the peak of the spike has been reached, the sodium channels thus begin to close, and the Na⁺ permeability is soon completely inactivated. At the same time, the K⁺ permeability of the membrane rises well above its resting value, and an outward movement of K⁺ takes place, eventually restoring the membrane potential to its original level. At the end of the spike the membrane has returned to the normal resting potential, but its Na⁺

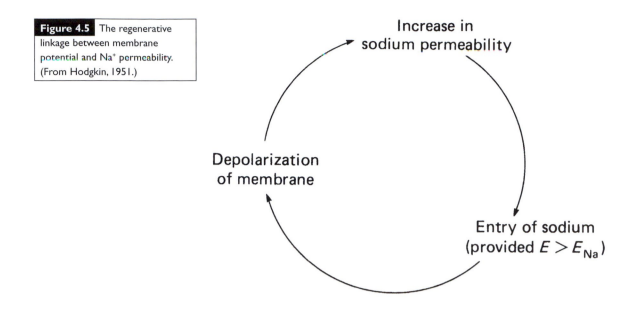

permeability mechanism is still inactivated. Lapse of further time allows the Na⁺ permeability to be reactivated, and hence restored to the quiescent state in which it is still very low, as is characteristic of the resting membrane, but is now ready once more to increase explosively if the system is retriggered.

According to this scheme, the most important features of the sodium channels are first that their opening is rapid and very steeply dependent on membrane potential, so that a relatively small degree of depolarization suffices to bring about a large rise in Na⁺ permeability (P_{Na}), and second that having opened quickly they are subject to a somewhat slower process of inactivation which closes them again even though the potential has not returned to its starting level, and may still be reversed. At least in the squid giant axon, the potassium channels are controlled just as strongly by the membrane potential, but their opening is delayed and they are not inactivated, the return of P_K to normal being wholly dependent on the repolarization of the membrane during the falling phase of the spike. The separation in time of the permeability changes, P_{Na} rising quickly and then being cut off by inactivation, while P_K only rises with an appreciable lag, helps to ensure that there is not too great an energetically wasteful interchange of Na⁺ and K⁺ at the peak of the spike unaccompanied by a useful alteration in the membrane potential. It may be noted that it is not essential to the conduction mechanism that P_K should increase at all. In the squid axon, the delayed rise of P_K enables the potential to return to normal faster than it otherwise would do, and so shortens the spike and speeds up conduction. But the inactivation of P_{Na} in conjunction with an unenhanced outflow of K⁺ ions would bring back the potential, albeit more slowly, and some types of nerve fibre are able to dispense with the rise of P_K.

4.3 | Voltage-clamp experiments

The increase in the Na^+ permeability of the membrane during the spike that is predicted by the sodium hypothesis can be measured with radioactive tracers by the method illustrated in Figure 4.4. But although this approach has the advantage of specificity, in that it provides unambiguous information about Na^+ movements and not those of any other ion, the time resolution of tracer experiments is rather poor, and the results refer only to the cumulative effect of a large number of impulses. In order to make a detailed study of the changes in membrane permeability in the course of a single action potential, it is necessary to resort to measurements of the electric current carried by the ions when they move across the membrane, which enable much greater sensitivity and much better time resolution to be achieved. However, the amount that can be learnt simply by recording the current that flows during the conducted action potential is very limited, because the permeability changes follow a fixed sequence determined by the nerve and not by the experimenter. To get around the difficulty, Hodgkin and Huxley exploited the approach originally due to Cole and Marmont in order to measure the ionic conductance of a nerve membrane whose potential was first 'clamped' at a chosen level and then subjected to a pre-determined series of abrupt changes. This enabled them to explore in considerable detail the laws governing the voltage-sensitive behaviour of the sodium and potassium channels, and present-day knowledge of the permeability mechanisms that underlie not only excitation and conduction in nerve and muscle, but also synaptic transmission, is derived very largely from *voltage-clamp* studies.

A typical experimental set-up for voltage-clamping a squid giant axon is shown in Figure 4.6. It requires the introduction of two internal electrodes, one for monitoring the potential at the centre of the stretch of axon to be clamped, and the other for passing current uniformly across the membrane over a somewhat greater length. In Hodgkin and Huxley's original apparatus, these electrodes were of the type seen in Figure 2.2, and were

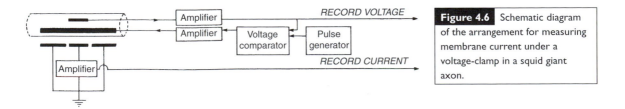

Figure 4.6 Schematic diagram of the arrangement for measuring membrane current under a voltage-clamp in a squid giant axon.

constructed by winding two spirals of AgCl-coated silver wire on a fine glass rod. Nowadays, the potential is generally recorded by a 50 μm micropipette filled with isotonic KCl (see Figure 2.1), to which is glued a platinum wire 75 μm in diameter whose terminal portion is left bare and platinized so that it will pass current without undue polarization. The external electrode consists of a platinized platinum sheet in three sections: the current flowing to the central section is amplified and recorded, while the two outer sections help to ensure the uniformity of clamping over the fully controlled region. After appropriate amplification, the internal potential is fed to a voltage comparator circuit, along with the square-wave signal to which it is to be clamped. The output from the comparator is applied to the internal current wire so as to increase or decrease the membrane current just enough to force the membrane potential to follow the square wave exactly. In electronic terms, this arrangement constitutes a negative-feedback control system in which the potential across the membrane is determined by the externally generated command signal, and the resulting membrane current is measured. In order to voltage-clamp smaller non-myelinated nerve fibres, single nerve cells, muscle fibres or the isolated node of Ranvier in a myelinated nerve fibre, various other electrode arrangements are called for, but the basic principle of the circuit remains the same.

The equivalent electrical circuit of the nerve membrane may be regarded, as shown in Figure 4.7, as a capacitance C_m connected in parallel with three resistive ionic pathways each incorporating a resistance (R_K, R_{Na} and R_{leak}) in series with a battery. For a given ionic pathway, the driving forces acting on the ions are the membrane potential E_m and the concentration gradient for that species of ion. As has been explained in Section 3.3, the concentration gradient may be equated with an electromotive force (e.m.f.) calculated from Equation (3.2) as the Nernst equilibrium potential, whence the appropriate values for the three battery potentials are E_K, E_{Na} and E_{leak}, and the net e.m.f. acting on each ion is the difference between E_m and its Nernst potential. It follows from Ohm's Law that the ionic currents I_K, I_{Na} and I_{leak} are given by

$$I_K = (E_m - E_K)/R_K \tag{4.1}$$

and so on. Although, in accordance with electrical convention, the ionic pathways are represented as resistances, it is often more convenient to think of them as the reciprocal conductances g_K, g_{Na} and g_{leak}. These represent the ease with which that particular ion can pass across the membrane, and are thus directly comparable with the permeability coefficients that appear in the constant field equation (see Section 3.3), though they are measured in different units. In the equivalent circuit, $R_K(= 1/g_K)$ and $R_{Na}(= 1/g_{Na})$ are indicated as being variable, and the object of voltage-clamp experiments is to investigate their dependence on membrane potential and time. R_{leak}, to which the main contributing ion is

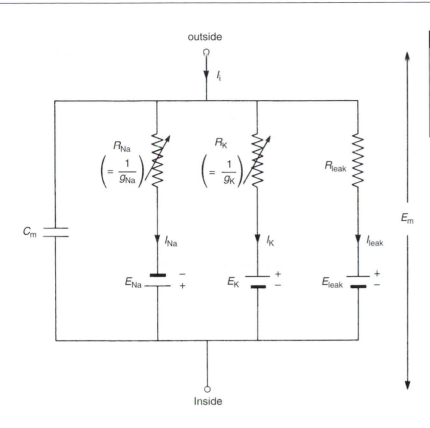

Cl^-, is constant. In the absence of externally applied current, the electrical model predicts that the value of E_m will be determined by the relative sizes of the ionic conductances. If g_K is, as in the resting condition, much larger than g_{Na}, E_m will lie close to E_K; but when the sodium channels are opened and g_{Na} rises, E_m will move towards E_{Na}. When the potential at which the membrane is clamped is suddenly altered, the current flowing across the membrane will consist of the capacity current required to charge or discharge C_m plus the ionic current that is to be measured. Hence the total current I will be given by

$$I = C_m \cdot [dE/dt] + I_i \qquad (4.2)$$

where I_i is the sum of the current flowing through all three ionic pathways. With a well-designed voltage-clamp system, $[dE/dt]$ should have fallen to zero and the flow of capacity current should therefore have ceased after no more than about 20 μs, so that all subsequent changes in the recorded current can be attributed to alterations in the Na^+ and K^+ conductances operative at the new membrane potential. Figure 4.8 shows a typical family of superimposed current records for a squid giant axon subjected to increasingly large voltage steps in the depolarizing direction. The initial capacity transients were too fast to be photographed, and what is seen is purely the ionic current. It is evident that there is an early phase of ionic current which flows inwards for small depolarizations and outwards for

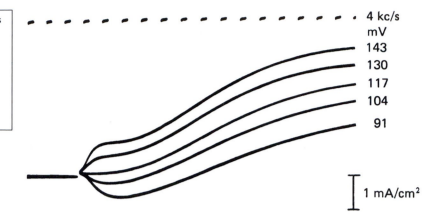

Figure 4.8 Membrane currents for large depolarizing voltage-clamp pulses; outward current upwards. The figures on the right show the change in internal potential in mV. Temperature 3.5 °C. (From Hodgkin (1958) after Hodgkin *et al.* (1952).)

large ones, and a late phase which is always outwards. This is consistent with the postulates of the sodium hypothesis, and next we have to consider how the contributions of I_{Na} and I_K can be separated from one another.

The method adopted by Hodgkin and Huxley for the analysis of their voltage-clamp records was to suppress the inward Na+ current by substituting choline for Na+ in the external medium. This procedure yielded records of the type shown in Figure 4.9, from which it is apparent that the removal of external Na+ converts the initial hump of inward current into an outward one, but has no effect on the late current, confirming that they are carried by Na+ and K+ ions, respectively. To eliminate the Na+ current completely, it was necessary to leave some Na+ in the external medium and to take E_m exactly to E_{Na}, where by definition $I_{Na} = 0$. In the experiment of Figure 4.10 this was achieved by reducing $[Na]_o$ to one-tenth and depolarizing by 56 mV; trace (*b*) shows the resulting record of the K+ current by itself. Subtraction of trace (*b*) from trace (*a*), which was recorded in normal sea water, then yielded trace (*c*) as the time course of the Na+ current. The currents thus measured were finally converted into conductances by taking $g_K = I_K/(E_m - E_K)$ and $g_{Na} = I_{Na}/(E_m - E_{Na})$. A plot of g_K and g_{Na} against time (Figure 4.11) shows that, as explained above, g_{Na} rises quickly and is then inactivated, while g_K rises with a definite lag and is not inactivated.

Separation of the two components of the ionic current can now be achieved more easily by recording the Na+ current after completely blocking the potassium channels, and vice versa. A good method of abolishing I_K is through the introduction of caesium into the axon by perfusion or dialysis: the Cs+ ions enter the mouths of the potassium channels from the inside, and block them very effectively. Figure 4.12 shows a typical family of I_{Na} records for voltage-clamp pulses of different sizes applied to a squid giant axon dialysed with caesium fluoride. For the sodium channels, a blocking agent is now available which acts externally at extremely

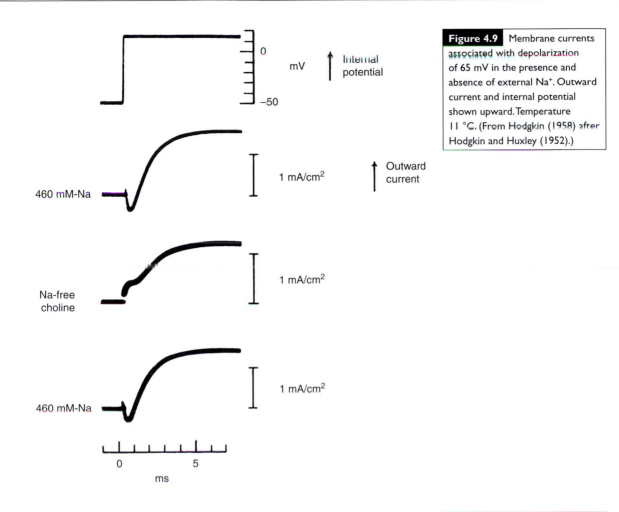

460 mM-Na

Na-free
choline

460 mM-Na

Figure 4.9 Membrane currents associated with depolarization of 65 mV in the presence and absence of external Na$^+$. Outward current and internal potential shown upward. Temperature 11 °C. (From Hodgkin (1958) after Hodgkin and Huxley (1952).)

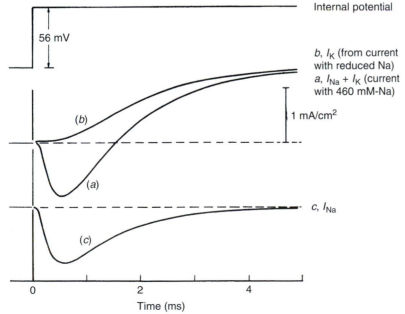

Internal potential

b, I_K (from current with reduced Na)
a, $I_{Na} + I_K$ (current with 460 mM-Na)

c, I_{Na}

Figure 4.10 Analysis of the ionic current changes in a squid giant axon during a voltage-clamp pulse that depolarized it by 56 mV. Trace (a) ($= I_{Na} + I_K$) shows the response with the axon in sea water containing 460 mM-Na. Trace (b) ($= I_K$) is the response with the axon in a solution made up of 10% sea water and 90% isotonic choline chloride solution. Trace (c) ($= I_{Na}$) is the difference between traces (a) and (b). Temperature 8.5 °C. (From Hodgkin (1958) after Hodgkin and Huxley (1952).)

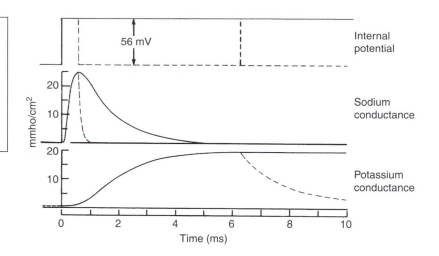

Figure 4.11 Time courses of the ionic conductance changes during a voltage-clamp pulse calculated from the current records shown in Figure 4.10. The dashed lines show the effect of repolarization after 0.6 or 6.3 ms. (From Hodgkin (1958) after Hodgkin and Huxley (1952).)

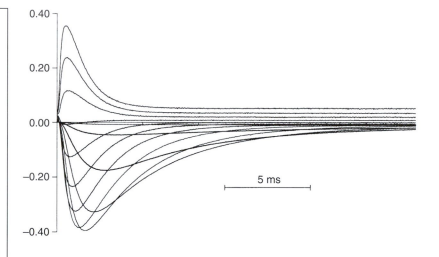

Figure 4.12 Superimposed traces of the Na⁺ current in a voltage-clamped squid axon whose potassium channels had been blocked by internal dialysis with 330 mM CsF + 20 mM NaF and which was bathed in a K-free artificial sea water containing 103 mM-NaCl and 421 mM-Tris buffer. The membrane was held at −70 mV and pulses were applied, taking the potential to levels varying between −40 and +80 mV in steps of 10 mV. Current scales mA/cm². For the smaller test pulses, the current flowed inward (downward), but above about +50 mV its direction reversed. For the largest pulses, inactivation was no longer complete, and the channels ended up in the non-inactivating open state. Temperature 5 °C. (Computer recording made by R. D. Keynes, N. G. Greeff, I. C. Forster and J. M. Bekkers.)

low concentrations, this being the Japanese puffer-fish poison tetrodotoxin, usually abbreviated to TTX, whose affinity constant for the Na⁺ sites is no more than about 3 nM. Figure 4.13 shows a family of I_K records for a squid axon dialysed with a potassium fluoride solution and bathed in a Na⁺-free solution containing 1 μM-TTX. A quantitative analysis of such records gives results identical with those obtained by Hodgkin and Huxley, and not only confirms their conclusions in every respect, but also provides convincing evidence for the validity of the assumption that the sodium and potassium channels are entirely separate entities between which the only connection is a strong dependence on a potential gradient common to both of them.

Hodgkin and Huxley next proceeded to devise a set of mathematical equations which would provide an empirical description of the behaviour of the Na⁺ and K⁺ conductances as a function of

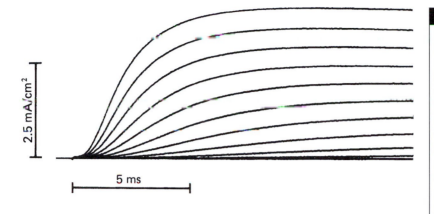

2.5 mA/cm²

5 ms

Figure 4.13 Superimposed traces of the potassium current in a voltage-clamped squid axon whose sodium channels had been blocked by bathing it in artificial sea water containing 1 µM-TTX, and which was dialysed internally with 350 mM-KF. The membrane was held at −70 mV, and pulses were applied, taking the potential to levels varying between −60 and +40 mV steps. Outward current is upward. Temperature 4 °C. (Computer recording made by R. D. Keynes, J. E. Kimura and N. G. Greeff.)

membrane potential and time. Thus the Na⁺ conductance was found to obey the relationship

$$g_{Na} = \bar{g}_{Na}\, m^3 h \qquad (4.3)$$

where $\bar{g}_{Na}$ is a constant representing the peak conductance attainable, m is a dimensionless activation parameter which varies between 0 and 1, and h is a similar inactivation parameter which varies between 1 and 0. The corresponding equation for the K⁺ conductance was

$$g_K = \bar{g}_K\, n^4 \qquad (4.4)$$

where $\bar{g}_K$ is the peak K⁺ conductance and n is another dimensionless activation parameter. The quantities m, h and n described the variation of the conductances with potential and time, and were determined by the differential equations describing first-order, unimolecular transitions between inactive and active states:

$$dm/dt = \alpha_m(1 - m) - \beta_m m \qquad (4.5)$$

$$dh/dt = \alpha_h(1 - h) - \beta_h h \qquad (4.6)$$

and $$dn/dt = \alpha_n(1 - n) - \beta_n n \qquad (4.7)$$

where the α and β terms are voltage-dependent rate constants whose dimensions are time⁻¹. The precise details of the voltage-dependence of the six rate constants need not concern us further, since Equations (4.3) to (4.7) have mainly been cited in order to help the mathematically minded reader to follow the steps that were necessary for the achievement of Hodgkin and Huxley's primary objective of testing the correctness of their description of the permeability system by calculating from their equations the shape of the propagated action potential.

The final step in Hodgkin and Huxley's arguments was thus the computation from data obtained under voltage-clamp conditions of the way in which the conducted action potential would be

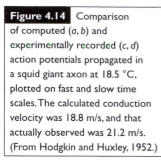

Figure 4.14 Comparison of computed (a, b) and experimentally recorded (c, d) action potentials propagated in a squid giant axon at 18.5 °C, plotted on fast and slow time scales. The calculated conduction velocity was 18.8 m/s, and that actually observed was 21.2 m/s. (From Hodgkin and Huxley, 1952.)

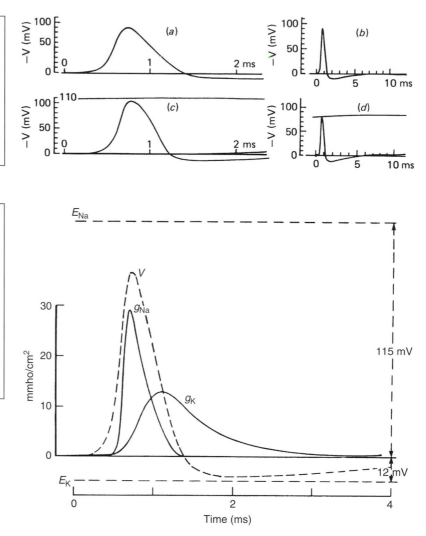

Figure 4.15 The time courses of the propagated action potential and underlying ionic conductance changes computed by Hodgkin and Huxley from their voltage-clamp data. The constants used were appropriate to a temperature of 18.5 °C. The calculated net entry of Na^+ was 4.33 pmole/cm^2, and the net exit of K^+ was 4.26 pmole/cm^2. Conduction velocity = 18.8 m/s. (From Hodgkin and Huxley, 1952.)

expected to behave. Figure 4.14 shows an example of the excellent agreement between the predicted time course of the propagated action potential at 18.5 °C and what was observed experimentally at this temperature. The velocity of conduction of the impulse could also be computed, and again the theoretical and observed values were satisfactorily close to one another. Lastly, the net exchange of Na^+ and K^+ could be predicted from the calculated extents and degree of overlap of the changes in g_{Na} and g_K during the spike that are illustrated in Figures 4.15 and 4.16. The total entry of sodium and the exit of potassium in a single impulse each worked out to be about 4.3 pmole/cm^2 membrane, which fits very well with the results of the analytical and tracer experiments discussed in Section 4.2. No more could have been asked of the sodium hypothesis than that it should have yielded, from purely electrical measurements, figures which checked so nicely with those based on a chemical approach.

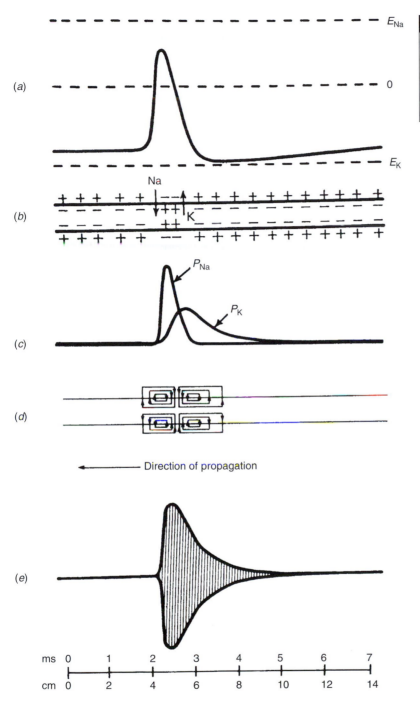

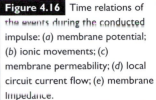

Figure 4.16 Time relations of the events during the conducted impulse: (a) membrane potential; (b) ionic movements; (c) membrane permeability; (d) local circuit current flow; (e) membrane impedance.

4.4 | Patch-clamp studies

Following the introduction by Neher and Sakmann (1976) of a voltage-clamp method for observing the currents flowing through single acetylcholine-receptor channels in denervated frog muscle

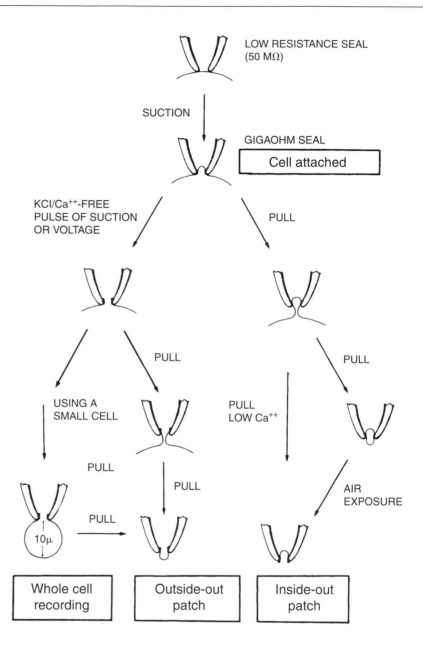

Figure 4.17 A schematic representation of the procedures for forming a gigaohm seal between the tip of a micropipette and a patch of cell membrane, and of achieving the recording configurations known as 'cell-attached', 'whole-cell', 'outside-out patch' and 'inside-out patch'. (From Hamill et al., 1981.)

LOW RESISTANCE SEAL (50 MΩ)

SUCTION

GIGAOHM SEAL

Cell attached

KCl/Ca++-FREE PULSE OF SUCTION OR VOLTAGE

PULL

USING A SMALL CELL

PULL

PULL LOW Ca++

PULL

PULL

AIR EXPOSURE

PULL

10μ

PULL

PULL

Whole cell recording

Outside-out patch

Inside-out patch

fibres (see Section 7.3.5), the technique of single-channel recording from a very small patch of membrane has been greatly extended (Figure 4.17), making it possible to study the properties of ion channels in every kind of living cell. The results of such studies are outside the scope of this volume, but it is clear that ion channels similar to those found in nerve and muscle have a variety of roles beyond the conduction of impulses in excitable tissues.

5

Voltage-gated ion channels

Both voltage-gated and ligand-gated ion channels are large protein molecules, as is the sodium pump Na,K-ATPase. In recent years the primary structure of a number of them has been determined, and by combining this information with the biophysical evidence, major advances have been made in our understanding of how they work at the molecular and submolecular levels.

5.1 | cDNA sequencing studies

A protein consists of a long chain built up of 20 different amino acids (Table 5.1), folded on itself in a rather complicated way. Its properties depend critically on the arrangement of the folds, which is determined by the exact order in which its constituent amino acids are strung together. This in turn is specified by the sequence of the nucleotide bases that make up the DNA molecules which constitute the genetic material of the cell. There are only four different bases, and each of the 20 amino acids corresponds according to a universally obeyed triplet code to a specific group of three of them. The information embodied in the base sequence of a DNA molecule is transcribed on to an intermediary messenger RNA, and is then translated during the synthesis of the protein to yield the correct sequence of amino acids. Rapid sequencing methods for nucleotides were perfected by Sanger and his colleagues, and modern recombinant DNA technology makes possible the cloning of DNA so that the quantity required for the determination can be prepared from a single gene. Hence the amino-acid sequences of proteins are nowadays most easily determined indirectly from the base sequences of the cDNA in which they are encoded.

5.2 | The primary structure of voltage-gated ion channels

The substantial voltages generated by the electric organ of the electric eel depend on the additive discharge of a large number of cells

Table 5.1 | *The amino acids found in proteins. Amino acids have the general formula R–CH(NH$_2$) COOH, where R is the side chain or residue. Proline is actually an imino acid, while cystine is two cysteines linked by a disulfide bridge. The standard abbreviations are given in three- and one-letter codes. The hydropathy index is taken from Kyte and Doolittle (1982)*

Type	Amino acid	Side chain	Abbreviations		Hydropathy index
Non-polar	Isoleucine	– CH(CH$_3$)CH$_2$.CH$_3$	Ile	I	4.5
	Valine	– CH(CH$_3$)$_2$	Val	V	4.2
	Leucine	– CH$_2$.CH(CH$_3$)$_2$	Leu	L	3.8
	Phenylalanine	– CH$_2$.C$_6$H$_5$	Phe	F	2.8
	Methionine	– CH$_2$.CH$_2$.SCH$_3$	Met	M	1.9
	Alanine	– CH$_3$	Ala	A	1.8
	Tryptophan	– CH$_2$C(CHNH)C$_6$H$_4$	Trp	W	−0.9
	Proline	– CH$_2$.CH$_2$.CH$_2^-$	Pro	P	−1.6
Uncharged Polar	Cysteine/cystine	– CH$_2$SH	Cys	C	2.5
	Glycine	– H	Gly	G	−0.4
	Threonine	– CH(OH)CH$_3$	Thr	T	−0.7
	Serine	– CH$_2$OH	Ser	S	−0.8
	Tyrosine	– CH$_2$C$_6$H$_4$OH	Tyr	Y	−1.3
	Histidine	– CH$_2$C(NHCHNCH)	His	H	−3.2
	Glutamine	– CH$_2$.CH$_2$.CO.NH$_2$	Gln	Q	−3.5
	Asparagine	– CH$_2$.CO.NH$_2$	Asn	N	−3.5
Acidic	Aspartic acid	– CH$_2$.COO$^-$	Asp	D	−3.5
	Glutamic acid	– CH$_2$CH$_2$COO$^-$	Glu	E	−3.5
Basic	Lysine	– (CH$_2$)$_4$.NH$_3^+$	Lys	K	−3.9
	Arginine	– (CH$_2$)$_3$NH.C(NH$_2$)=NH$_3^+$	Arg	R	−4.5

that are derived embryonically from muscle (see Figure 2.4g). Their electrical excitability involves an increase of Na$^+$ permeability in the usual way, and this type of electric organ therefore provided ideal material, first for isolating and purifying the sodium channel protein and then for enabling its amino-acid sequence to be determined. The initial biochemistry was greatly facilitated by the fact that the protein could be labelled with high specificity by the Japanese puffer-fish poison tetrodotoxin (TTX). The sodium channel was shown to be a single large peptide with a molecular mass of about 260 kDa, which is glycosylated at several points on incorporation into the membrane.

A team of scientists led by Numa and Noda at Kyoto University successfully cloned and sequenced the cDNA of the sodium channel both in the *Electrophorus* electric organ and in rat brain. This was quickly followed up elsewhere by the cloning of voltage-gated potassium channels, most notably the *Shaker* gene of the fruit fly *Drosophila*, and of voltage-gated calcium channels such as the dihydropyridine receptor in muscle (see Section 10.6). It has now become clear that

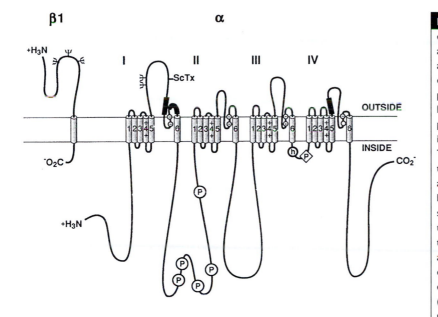

Figure 5.1 Primary structures of the α- and β1-subunits of a sodium channel illustrated as transmembrane folding diagrams. The bold lines are polypeptide chains with the length of each segment roughly proportional to its true length in a rat brain sodium channel. The cylinders represent probable transmembrane α-helices, and parts of the external links between transmembrane segments S5 and S6 are shown as tucked back into the membrane to form the external pore. Sites are indicated of experimentally demonstrated glycosylation ψ, cAMP-dependent phosphorylation (P in a circle), protein kinase C phosphorylation (P in a diamond), amino-acid residues required for TTX binding (ScTx), and of the inactivation particle (h in a circle). (From Catterall (1992) with permission of the American Physiological Society.

there is a large family of membrane proteins selective for K⁺, Na⁺ or Ca²⁺ ions, and gated not only by voltage, but also in a variety of other ways, whose primary structures are all closely related. Taking the *Electrophorus* sodium channel as the prototype, the protein is a large monomer containing 1820 amino-acid residues. The α-subunit shown diagrammatically in Figure 5.1 can, when expressed on its own, produce a normally functioning sodium channel. It consists of four homologous domains labelled I, II, III and IV that span the membrane, and which have closely similar amino-acid sequences. The size and structure of calcium channels are much the same, as are potassium channels, except that they are tetramers built up of four identical domains.

Of the 20 possible amino acids that make up a protein, it may be seen in Table 5.1 that the residues of eight are non-polar, seven are polar but uncharged, two are acidic and carry a negative charge, and three are basic and positively charged. The non-polar residues are hydrophobic, and therefore tend to be located in the centre of the molecule in the lipid core of the membrane. The polar or charged residues are hydrophilic, and are more likely to be found in the aqueous environment of the cytoplasm or at the outer surface of the membrane. From a study of what is known as the hydropathy index of different stretches of the amino-acid chain it has been deduced that each of the homologous domains comprises six segments that are largely hydrophobic and form α-helices crossing the membrane from one side to the other. These segments are represented as cylinders in Figure 5.1. The amino-acid sequences of segments S2, S3 and S4 in the voltage-gated sodium and potassium channels of some typical species are shown in Figure 5.2. Those of voltage-gated calcium channels are very similar.

Figure 5.2 The amino-acid sequences of the charge-carrying S2, S3 and S4 transmembrane segments of all four domains of voltage-gated K⁺ channels, and of the individual domains of Na⁺ channels, for the squid *Loligo opalescens*, the fly *Drosophila* and rat brain. Positively charged arginine residues (**R**) and lysine residues (**K**) are in bold type and the stretches over which they are separated by two non-polar residues are underlined. Negatively charged residues of aspartate (**D**) and glutamate (**E**) are ringed. (Data selected from Figures 1, 3 and 4 of Keynes and Elinder, 1999.)

inside   outside

		Sequence	Species
K⁺	S2	C S A F **R** I L L Ⓔ M T F W I I C G T Ⓔ I I	*Loligo* sKv1A
		C A L F **R** V T L Ⓔ F T F W I I C L T Ⓔ I L	*Drosophila* Shaker
		C A F F **R** V V L Ⓔ F S F W I I C L T Ⓔ V I	Rat rKv1.1
Na⁺	IS2	**R** A F L **K** I L A Ⓔ C T Y I G T F I W Ⓔ S V	*Loligo* sNa2
		K A I I **K** I V M Ⓔ I S Y I A L F I Y Ⓔ A Ⓔ	*Drosophila* dNa1
		R A L I **K** I L S Ⓔ F T Y I G T F T Y Ⓔ V N	Rat rNaB2
	IIS2	L A L I **K** L F A Ⓔ A A F V A T F V Y N G I	*Loligo* sNa2
		L A M L **K** V I C Ⓔ F T F I S T F V **K** N G V	*Drosophila* dNa1
		M A I I **K** L F M Ⓔ A T F I G T F V L N G V	Rat rNaB2
	IIIS2	F A F W **K** I F M Ⓔ G I F I V T F C **K** Ⓓ M Y	*Loligo* sNa2
		L A L W **K** L I M Ⓔ V V F I L C F S F N I W	*Drosophila* dNa1
		Y A V W **K** L L M Ⓔ L I F I Y T F V **K** Ⓓ A Y	Rat rNaB2
	IVS2	L G M L **K** M V C Ⓔ G T F I G I F V M N I Y	*Loligo* sNa2
		L G V I **K** V I A Ⓔ L G F V T T F F A N S V	*Drosophila* dNa1
		L S I L **K** L V C Ⓔ G T F L V I F V L N I W	Rat rNaB2
K⁺	S3	S M N A I Ⓓ V V S I M P Y F I T L G T V I	*Loligo* sKv1A
		V M N V I Ⓓ I I A I I P Y F I T L A T V V	*Drosophila* Shaker
		I M N F I Ⓓ I V A I I P Y F I T L G T Ⓔ I	Rat rKv1.1
Na⁺	IS3	A W N W L Ⓓ F V V I G L A Y L T Ⓔ V V Ⓓ L	*Loligo* sNa2
		P W N W L Ⓓ F V V I T M R Y A T I G M Ⓔ V	*Drosophila* dNa1
		P W N W L Ⓓ F T V I T F A Y V T Ⓔ F V N L	Rat rNaB2
	IIS3	P W N V F Ⓓ S F I V F L S M L Ⓔ L G L G G	*Loligo* sNa2
		G W N I F Ⓓ L L I V T A S L L Ⓓ I I F Ⓔ L	*Drosophila* dNa1
		G W N I F Ⓓ G F I V S L S L M Ⓔ L G L A N	Rat rNaB2
	IIIS3	A W C W L Ⓓ F L I V A V S I I M L A A Ⓔ S	*Loligo* sNa2
		F W T I L Ⓓ F I I V F V S V F S L L I Ⓔ Ⓔ	*Drosophila* dNa1
		A W C W L Ⓓ F L I V D V S L V S L T A N A	Rat rNaB2
	IVS3	P W N I F Ⓓ F V V V V L S I L G I A L S Ⓓ	*Loligo* sNa2
		P W N S P Ⓓ F L L V L A S I L G I L M Ⓔ Ⓓ	*Drosophila* dNa1
		G W N I F Ⓓ F V V V I L S I V G M F L A Ⓔ	Rat rNaB2
K⁺	S4	Q L G **K** S H **R** S L **K** F I **R** F V **R** V L **R** I V **R** L	*Loligo* sKv1A
		Q L G **K** S H **R** S L **K** F I **R** F V **R** V L **R** I V **R** L	*Drosophila* Shaker
		Q L G **K** S H **R** S L **K** F I **R** F V **R** V L **R** I V **R** L	Rat rKv1.1
Na⁺	IS4	**K** L G P I V A V T **K** L A **R** L V **R** F T **R** L A S L	*Loligo* sNa2
		K L G P M I S V T **K** L A **R** L V **R** F T **R** L G A L	*Drosophila* dNa1
		K L G P I V S I T **K** L A **R** L V **R** F T **R** L A S V	Rat rNaB2
	IIS4	N L T P W S **K** A L **K** F V **R** L L **R** F S **R** L V S L	*Loligo* sNa2
		K M T T W S **K** A L **K** L A **R** L L **R** L G **R** L V S L	*Drosophila* dNa1
		N L T P W S **K** A L **K** F V **R** L L **R** F S **R** L V S L	Rat rNaB2
	IIIS4	**R** M G Ⓔ S **R** S V A **R** L P **R** L A **R** L T **R** M S **R** F	*Loligo* sNa2
		R M G Q W **R** S I A **R** L P **R** L A **R** L T **R** L S **R** L	*Drosophila* dNa1
		R M G Ⓔ F **R** S L A **R** L P **R** L A **R** L T **R** L S **K** I	Rat rNaB2
	IVS4	**R** I G **K** A S **K** V L **R** L V **R** G V **R** F G **R** V V **R** L	*Loligo* sNa2
		R I G **K** A A **K** I L **R** L I **R** G I **R** F V **R** V V **R** L	*Drosophila* dNa1
		R I G **K** A G **K** I L **R** L I **R** G I **R** A L **R** I V **R** F	Rat rNaB2

A specific requirement of the channels with which this chapter is concerned is that the structure should incorporate voltage-sensing elements that will respond to alterations in the electric field across the membrane. The best candidates to act as voltage sensors are agreed to be the S4 segments whose sequences are shown in Figure 5.2, which are capable of moving across the membrane to a limited extent in a screwlike fashion. Each one carries between four and eight positively charged arginine or lysine residues, always separated by a pair of non-polar or in a few cases uncharged polar residues. They operate as explained below in conjunction with segments S2 and S3, on which are located altogether three negatively charged aspartate or glutamate residues in fixed positions.

An inevitable limitation of cDNA sequencing studies is that although they provide a wealth of accurate information about the primary structure of membrane proteins, it is necessary to depend on indirect and often speculative arguments to decide exactly how the molecule is folded, and to elucidate the nature of the conformational changes that bring about the opening and closing of the channels.

An additional tool that is particularly valuable in the study of voltage-gated and ligand-gated ion channels is the ability to express the proteins whose primary structures have been determined, by the injection of the corresponding messenger RNA into the oocytes of the African clawed toad *Xenopus*. These are large cells that are about to develop into mature eggs. They possess the normal translation machinery, and will respond to the injection of messenger RNA by making the protein for which it codes and incorporating it in the membrane. After synthesizing the corresponding messenger RNA, the majority of the voltage-gated and ligand-gated channel proteins that have so far been isolated have been successfully expressed in such oocytes, and have been shown either by patch-clamping or by recording macroscopic single-cell currents to behave in an essentially normal fashion. An important extension of the technique is then to alter the sequence of the amino-acid residues by the procedure known as site-directed mutagenesis to explore in detail the effect of artificial modifications of the protein structure.

5.3 | The sodium gating current

An essential avenue towards a detailed understanding of the mode of operation of voltage-gated ion channels is to investigate the kinetics of the macroscopic ion currents in the manner adopted in the classical paper of Hodgkin and Huxley (1952). However, such studies are in one respect limited in their scope, because they throw light only on the kinetics of the open state, and reveal relatively little about the series of closed states through which the system must certainly pass during activation and inactivation.

It was pointed out by Hodgkin and Huxley that the voltage-dependence of the sodium conductance implies that the gating mechanism itself is charged, and further that whenever a change in membrane potential operates the gate, there must be a movement down the electric field of the charged side groups that it carries, giving rise to a displacement current that necessarily precedes the flow of ion current. The *asymmetry current* or *gating current*, as it has come to be called, remained undetected for some years because the corresponding transfer of charge within the membrane is so small compared with the transfer of ions across it. However, in 1973/4, Keynes and Rojas at Plymouth, and Armstrong and Bezanilla working at Woods Hole, succeeded in recording an asymmetrical component of the Na^+ current in voltage-clamped squid axons. To achieve this, it was first necessary to block the passage of Na^+ ions through the open sodium channels by bathing the axon in an Na^+-free solution containing a high concentration of TTX, which fortunately turned

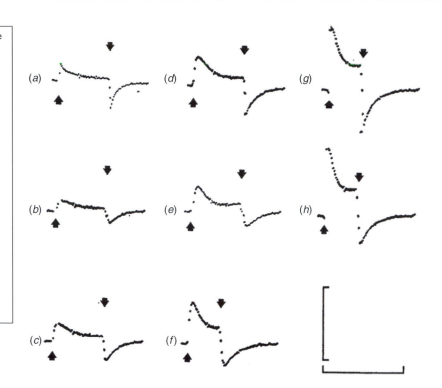

Figure 5.3 Early records of the sodium gating currents in squid axons made by Keynes and Rojas (1974). The external solution was Na⁺-, K⁺- and Mg²⁺-free artificial sea water containing 300 nM saxitoxin and the axon was perfused with 55 mM caesium fluoride. For each record, 60 depolarizing and hyperpolarizing pulses, starting and finishing at the arrows, were applied at a frequency of 2 s⁻¹ and were averaged. Pulse amplitude, (a–h), 40–110 mV. Resting membrane potential −52 mV, holding potential −70 mV. Temperature 7 °C. Vertical bar 5.56 μA; horizontal bar 2500 μs. (From Keynes and Rojas, 1974.)

out to seal up the channel at its mouth without interfering with the operation of the voltage-gate. The K⁺ channels were also blocked by perfusion or internal dialysis with a caesium or tetramethylammonium fluoride solution. The symmetrical capacity transient that arises when charging or discharging the passive membrane capacity was eliminated electronically. These analysis procedures yielded the first records representing sodium gating currents typified in Figure 5.3.

Although gating currents have since been recorded at the node of Ranvier, in various other types of nerve and muscle, and in sodium and potassium channels expressed in *Xenopus* oocytes, the preparation that enables the best possible time resolution to be achieved is still the squid giant axon. Even so, some 20 years elapsed before the kinetics of the sodium gating current could be seen to fit satisfactorily with those of the ion currents and be readily interpreted in terms of the molecular structure of the channel. The recordings in Figure 5.4a show that although for the most negative test pulses the current rises quickly and decays exponentially, for the pulse to −17 mV a small delayed rise can clearly be seen to come in just after the start of the relaxation. For larger pulses the slowly rising phase becomes increasingly prominent, reaching its peak with a roughly constant delay of about 30 μs. This initial part of the gating current is probably generated by the first two transitions in the four S4 units operating in parallel. The trace (b) shows that the rise of Na⁺ current itself begins only around 75 μs after the start of the test

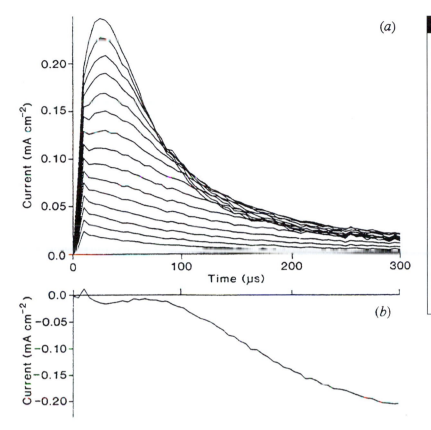

(a)

(b)

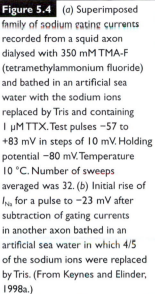

Figure 5.4 (a) Superimposed family of sodium gating currents recorded from a squid axon dialysed with 350 mM TMA-F (tetramethylammonium fluoride) and bathed in an artificial sea water with the sodium ions replaced by Tris and containing 1 μM TTX. Test pulses −57 to +83 mV in steps of 10 mV. Holding potential −80 mV. Temperature 10 °C. Number of sweeps averaged was 32. (b) Initial rise of I_{Na} for a pulse to −23 mV after subtraction of gating currents in another axon bathed in an artificial sea water in which 4/5 of the sodium ions were replaced by Tris. (From Keynes and Elinder, 1998a.)

pulse, so that the two activating steps are nearly complete before the third and final step opens the channel. These findings have at last provided a satisfactory basis for relating the kinetics of the gating current to the kinetics of the open state, and to the structure of the channel and other experimental evidence.

5.4 | The screw-helical mechanism of voltage-gating

It is clear from the structural studies that every voltage-gated ion channel incorporates four voltage sensors that operate in parallel, there being, as shown in Figure 5.2, an identical one in each domain of the tetrameric potassium channels. In the monomeric sodium channels there are four sensors that vary between four and eight in the number of positive charges carried in the individual domains, while the members of the related family of calcium channels, not shown in Figure 5.2, carry four or five charges. In order for a single channel to be opened, it is agreed from measurements on *Shaker* K⁺ channels, and also on sodium channels from squid axons and from non-inactivating skeletal muscle fibres expressed in oocytes, that 12 or slightly more electronic charges (e_0) have to be transferred, so that the transfer brought about by each S4 unit is $3e_0$. Careful measurements of gating-charge kinetics in squid axons have shown that each separate step in the opening, inactivation and late re-opening of the channels involves just $1e_0$ and no more. Studies of gating-current noise in *Shaker* K^+ channels and sodium channels expressed in oocytes have suggested the existence of 'single shots' of current carrying $2.3e_0$ accompanied by others carrying a single charge, but these extra-large pulses do not appear to be created by a single voltage sensor, and may rather be related to the phenomenon of re-opening in the inactivated state that must next be discussed.

It was discovered by Chandler and Meves in 1970 in squid axons that in their inactivated steady state, sodium channels could sometimes be observed to re-open briefly. This behaviour was later observed in other species, though in no case was its precise function obvious. In 1993, Keynes and Meves carried out a careful study at Plymouth of the probability functions (PF) both for the normal openings and for the subsequent delayed re-openings, as may be seen in Figure 5.5.

These observations demonstrated clearly that the equilibrium potential for the re-opening was as much as 100 mV more positive than the potential for the normal opening, which suggested that two different voltage sensors were involved. This was borne out by the facts that the ionic permeability of the individual channels when re-opened was less than half as great in the inactivated state than in the initial open state, and that the temperature coefficient was much larger for the initial opening than in the inactivated state,

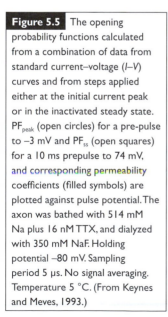

Figure 5.5 The opening probability functions calculated from a combination of data from standard current–voltage (I–V) curves and from steps applied either at the initial current peak or in the inactivated steady state. PF_{peak} (open circles) for a pre-pulse to −3 mV and PF_{ss} (open squares) for a 10 ms prepulse to 74 mV, and corresponding permeability coefficients (filled symbols) are plotted against pulse potential. The axon was bathed with 514 mM Na plus 16 nM TTX, and dialyzed with 350 mM NaF. Holding potential −80 mV. Sampling period 5 μs. No signal averaging. Temperature 5 °C. (From Keynes and Meves, 1993.)

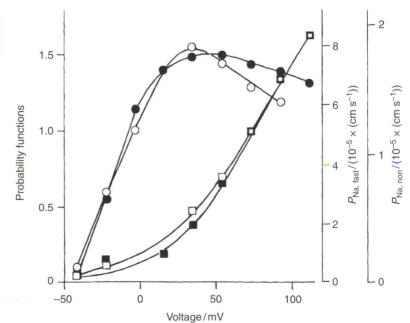

when the Q_{10} was close to unity. There is as yet no evidence as to the precise identity of the second voltage sensor that brings about the re-opening of the sodium channels, nor as to where it is located and how the two voltage sensors are appropriately linked together. But a number of types of one-domain voltage-gated ion channel selective for K^+, Na^+ or Ca^{2+} are now well known to be found in bacteria. These include the sodium channel NaChBac described by Catterall (2001), and one of them might be involved.

The screw-helical theory of voltage-gating put forward in 1986 by Catterall, Guy and others suggested that the positive charges located in every third position on S4 were arranged on the α-helix as a spiral ribbon, and in the resting state were paired with fixed negative charges on neighbouring helices. When a depolarization of the membrane increased the outward force acting on the positive charges, the S4 helix was free to undergo a screw-like motion by rotating through 60° and moving 0.45 nm outwards, so that each movable positive charge could proceed to pair up with the next fixed negative charge. Such a movement would bring an unpaired positive charge to the outer surface of the membrane, and at the same time would create an unpaired negative charge at the inner surface, so transferring approximately one electronic charge outwards. By twisting three times in succession through 60°, each S4 segment could therefore transfer a total of $3e_0$, as is observed.

This proposition meets with difficulty if the hydrophobic central pore extends across the whole thickness of the membrane, because there are more positive charges on the S4 segments than negative charges on the other five transmembrane segments to pair up with them. However, the elegant studies on the accessibility of the S4 charges to hydrophilic reagents on both sides of the membrane, carried out by Yang et al. (1996) on sodium channels, and by Larsson et al. (1996) on Shaker K^+ channels, have demonstrated that the hydrophobic section of the central pore must be appreciably shorter than was originally thought. Taking this into account, the purely diagrammatic picture in Figure 5.6 shows the stages in the positions of the mobile S4 segments in order to be paired successively with one of the fixed negative charges. Their completion would be followed allosterically by further conformational changes that are electrically

Figure 5.6 A strictly diagrammatic representation of the screw-helical outward movement of the positive charges carried by S4 in a Shaker K^+ channel. Each outward step transfers one electronic charge from its position on the α-helix inside the cell to the external solution. The three negative charges shown on the left occupy fixed positions on S2 and S3, and salt bridges are formed with two of the positive charges in the closed hyperpolarized state and three in the intermediate and open states. (From Keynes and Elinder, 1999.)

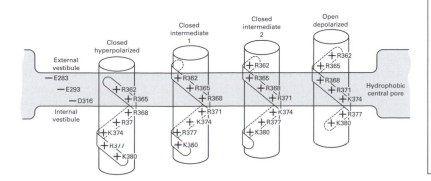

invisible and finally open the channels themselves, possibly located between segments S5 and S6.

A vitally important feature of the system is certainly that the individual steps made by the voltage sensors are stabilized by the formation of salt bridges between three of the movable positive charges and three fixed negative charges located on segments S2 and S3. As may be seen in Figure 5.2, two of the negative charges are located respectively nine places from the inner end of S2 and six places from the inner end of S3, while the third ones are more widely scattered near the outer ends of S2 or S3. There is evidence from several sources for the occurrence in the open state of ion pairing between the particular residues shown in Figure 5.2, while a modelling exercise has shown that these interactions would be geometrically compatible with a structure in which S2 and S3 are parallel α-helices, while S4 is another α-helix tilted to cross them at an angle.

Methods for determining the exact structures of the system in its transient intermediate states are not yet available, but an alternative manner in which the electric field produced by the S4 segments may be shifted appreciably by the movement of aqueous crevices in the channel protein has recently been established by Ahern and Horn (2005) in experiments on *Shaker* K$^+$ channels. It has moreover now been elegantly shown by Broomand and Elinder (2008) that the positively charged S4 segment is indeed suitably tilted so as to be free to slide and rotate in order to make electrostatic contacts with negative channels in S2 and S3, as shown in Figure 5.6. Although there is still no generally agreed answer on the problem, the consensus is thus converging on a screw-helical model in which both S4 and its environs rearrange dynamically as charge moves, without moving through more than a fraction of a nanometre. A powerful argument in its support is that it fits nicely with the nearly perfect conservation of the location of the negative charges in the sequences of S2 and S3 in every voltage-gated ion channel, whether selective for K$^+$, Na$^+$ or Ca^{2+}, across the entire animal kingdom. It follows that at least in sodium channels, the S4 segments may be regarded as wriggling about appreciably during their opening.

It is now accepted that, unlike those in squid that inactivate only very slowly, there are other types of potassium channel that display a rapid but voltage-independent inactivation. Nevertheless, in sodium channels the process of inactivation, as well as activation is apparently voltage dependent and is perhaps controlled primarily by voltage sensor IVS4 acting in conjunction with the internal link between domains III and IV seen in Figure 5.1. In order to account for the extra length of IVS4, inactivation might involve a fourth transfer of $1e_0$ in this voltage sensor accompanied by another undefined conformational change affecting the hydration pathway of the central activation gate. A fifth transfer of a single charge could then bring about delayed re-openings of the channel that account for the small inward flow of Na current taking place during the inactivated steady state.

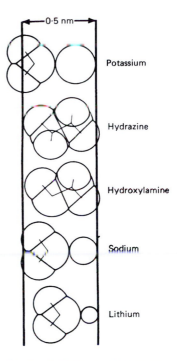

5.5 | The ionic selectivity of voltage-gated channels

Another essential feature is that every type of ion channel should be capable of a marked discrimination in favour of Na+, K+ or Ca2+ ions. Appropriate selectivity filters are invariably located in an extracellular pore region of the channel into which are tucked the four links between the outer ends of the S5 and S6 segments.

In the case of the sodium channel, Hille (1971) has concluded from studies of its relative permeability at the node of Ranvier to certain small organic cations, that selection depends on a good fit between the dimensions of the penetrating ion and those of the mouth of the channel. As indicated in Figure 5.7, only molecules measuring less than about 0.3 by 0.5 nm in cross-section are able to pass the filter. However, there were striking differences in permeability between some cations whose sizes were the same. Thus hydroxylamine ($OH-NH_3^+$) and hydrazine ($NH_2-NH_3^+$) readily entered the channel, but methylamine ($CH_3-NH_3^+$) did not. In order to explain the discrepancy, Hille proposed that the sodium channel is lined at its narrowest point with carbonyl oxygen atoms. Positively charged ions containing hydroxyl (OH) or amino (NH_2) groups are able to pass through the channel by making hydrogen bonds with the oxygens, but those containing methyl (CH_3) groups are excluded by their inability to form hydrogen bonds. The geometry of the situation is such that Na+ ions can divest themselves of all but one of their shell of water molecules by interacting with the strategically placed oxygen atoms, and the energy barrier that they encounter is therefore relatively low. The same is true for Li+, but the somewhat larger K+ ions cannot shed their hydration shell as easily, making P_K for the sodium channel only one twelfth as great as P_{Na}.

Calcium channels are normally permeable to Sr2+ and Ba2+ ions, but completely impermeable to monovalent cations. When, however, external [Ca2+] is greatly reduced, the channels become permeable to both K+ and Na+ ions. It is therefore thought that the calcium channel has two high-affinity Ca2+ binding sites at its mouth, and that if neither is occupied, monovalent ions can readily enter, while if one is occupied, Na+ and K+ ions are effectively kept out by electrostatic repulsion. When both sites are occupied, the flow both of divalent and monovalent cations rises again.

It was supposed some years ago that with a constant potential difference across the membrane, the chance of any individual K+ ion crossing the membrane in a given time interval would be unaffected by the other ions that were present, as it was for Na+ ions. But in some experiments that Hodgkin and Keynes had been doing

Figure 5.7 Scale drawings showing the effective sizes of Li+, Na+ and K+ ions, each with one molecule of water, and of unhydrated hydroxylamine and hydrazine ions. The vertical lines 0.5 nm apart represent the postulated space between oxygen atoms available for cations able to pass through the sodium channel. Methylamine would look just like hydrazine in this kind of picture, but is nevertheless unable to enter the channel. (After Hille, 1971.)

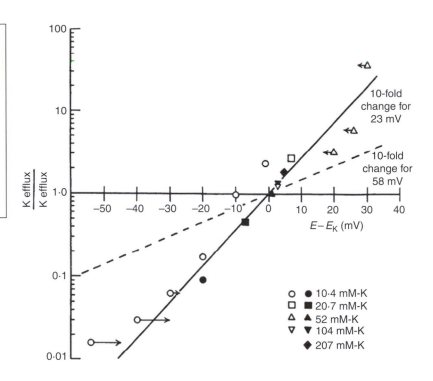

Figure 5.8 The effect of the electrical driving force $E - E_K$, on the potassium flux ratio in *Sepia* axons. The filled-in symbols are based on flux measurements using 17–29 mm lengths of fibre in the absence of applied current, and the other points were obtained with axons mounted for the application of current. The arrows show approximate corrections for cable effects. (From Hodgkin and Keynes, 1955b).

in 1953 on the movements of K⁺ ions in *Sepia* giant axons, reason was found to suspect that the dependence of the fluxes on potassium concentrations and membrane potential was misbehaving in some way. Experiments were therefore carried out by Hodgkin and Keynes (1955b) to measure the dependence of the potassium flux ratios between ion influx and efflux, systematically against the driving force $E - E_K$, with the results shown in Figure 5.8.

On the assumption that K⁺ ions do move in a wholly independent fashion across the membrane, it can readily be shown that the flux ratio would exhibit a 10-fold change for a 58 mV change in the value of $E - E_K$ where E is the membrane potential and E_K is the equilibrium potential for K⁺. But what was observed experimentally in axons poisoned with DNP to abolish the sodium efflux was a signficiantly greater change of 10 times for only 23 mV. This large departure from the independence relation could best be explained by assuming that K⁺ ions tend to move through the membrane in narrow channels which constrained them to move in single file, and there should, on average, be several ions in a channel at any moment.

The explanation that the K⁺ ions were constrained in some way to pass through the nerve membrane in single file was quickly accepted, and the simple mechanical model shown in Figure 5.9a was constructed by Hodgkin and Keynes (1955b) to test it. It consisted of two circular chambers, each containing a number of steel balls, connected by a pore just wide enough to allow a ball to pass through it, whose length could be increased to contain three balls

(a)

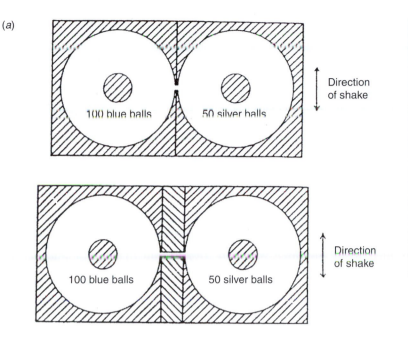

Direction of shake

Direction of shake

Figure 5.9 (a) The mechanical model used by Hodgkin and Keynes (1955b) to mimic their K⁺ flux data from *Sepia* axons. Single-filing of the exchange of ball bearings between the two compartments took place only when the chambers were connected by a pore long enough to contain three balls at a time, and too narrow for the balls to bypass one another. (Reproduced with permission.) (b) The similar structure of the filter in the pore of bacterial potassium channels, as described by Doyle *et al.* (1998) and McCleskey (1999).

(b)

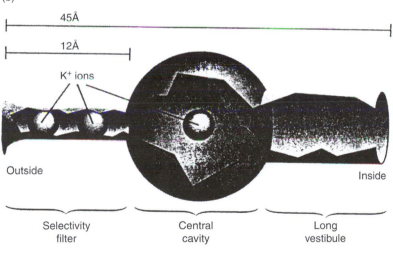

at a time. 100 balls that had been blued by heating were put in the left-hand chamber and 50 balls, identical except in being silver in colour, were put in the right-hand chamber. When shaken vigorously by a motor for 15 s, the balls rattled about with a random 'Brownian' movement, and a certain number passed through the pore. The number of blue balls which moved from left to right was counted, and compared with the number of silver balls which had moved in the opposite direction during the same time interval. The experiments were repeated a number of times to check that there were no slight asymmetries or tilt of the apparaus, and no differences between the two sets of balls, and the results were averaged.

The first successful X-ray crystallographical study of any part of an ion channel was carried out by Doyle *et al.* (1998) on the structure of the potassium filter in bacterial K^+ channels and later confirmed by Jiang *et al.* (2003) and also reviewed by Gulbis and Doyle (2004). The existence of an appreciable number of potassium channels with a variety of structures and functions is now recognized and it is clear that in the voltage-dependent channel KvAP of *Shaker* nerves, the four S5–S6 links create an inverted cone cradling the narrow select-ivity filter of the pore, 1.2 nm in length, at its outer end. Here the main-chain atoms create a stack of sequential carbonyl oxygen rings, providing sites energetically suitable to be substituted for the hydra-tion shell of a K^+ ion. Above and below this narrow section of the K^+ filter, the pore is somewhat wider so that the hydrated K^+ ions are free to move on, while just two naked K^+ ions can be fitted into the filter itself, although within it they cannot bypass one another. In every type of potassium channel, however it is gated, cDNA sequen-cing reveals the presence of an identically structured selectivity filter. The simple collision theory derived by Hodgkin and Keynes (1955b) to explain single-file diffusion of K^+ ions in *Sepia* axons has therefore turned out to be precisely in line with the actual structure, and their crude mechanical model with ball bearings rattling about in two compartments connected by a narrow passage is remarkably close to a greatly scaled-up version of the filter designed by Nature perhaps a billion years ago.

Cable theory and saltatory conduction

6.1 | The spread of potential changes in a cable system

The propagation of the nervous impulse depends not only on the electrical excitability of the nerve membrane, but also on the *cable structure* of the nerve. We have already seen that the passive electrical properties of a patch of membrane can be represented as a capacitance C_m in parallel with a resistance R_m, so that the circuit diagram of a length of axon is the network shown in Figure 6.1, where R_o is the longitudinal resistance of the external medium, and R_i is the longitudinal resistance of the axoplasm. Such a network is typical of a sheathed electric cable, albeit one with rather poor insulation, because R_m is not nearly as large compared with R_i as it would be if the conducting core were a metal. If a constant current is passed transversely across the membrane so as to set up a potential difference V_o between inside and outside at one point, then the voltage elsewhere will fall off with the distance x in the manner indicated in the lower part of Figure 6.1. The law governing this passive *electrotonic* spread of potential is

$$V_x = V_o \, e^{-x/\lambda} \tag{6.1}$$

where the *space constant* λ is given by

$$\lambda^2 = R_m/(R_o + R_i) \tag{6.2}$$

A similar argument applies in the case of a brief pulse of current, except that the value of C_m then has to be taken into account in addition to that of R_m. However, it is not necessary to enter here into the detailed mathematics of the passive spread of potential in a cable system, and it will suffice to note that theory and experiment are in good agreement.

Suppose now that an action potential of amplitude V_o has been set up over a short length of axon, and that the threshold-potential change necessary to stimulate the resting membrane is a certain fraction, say one-fifth of V_o. Because of the cable structure of the

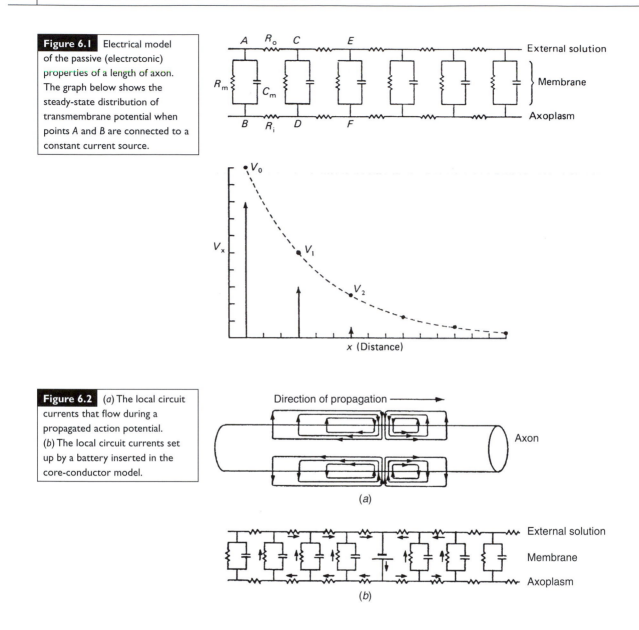

Figure 6.1 Electrical model of the passive (electrotonic) properties of a length of axon. The graph below shows the steady-state distribution of transmembrane potential when points *A* and *B* are connected to a constant current source.

Figure 6.2 (*a*) The local circuit currents that flow during a propagated action potential. (*b*) The local circuit currents set up by a battery inserted in the core-conductor model.

nerve, current will flow in local circuits on either side of the active region, as indicated in Figure 6.2, and the depolarization will spread passively. At a critical distance in front of the active region, which with the assumption made above would be about 1.5 times the space constant, the amount of depolarization will just exceed the threshold. This part of the axon will then become active in its turn, and the active region will move forwards. Provided that the axon is uniform in diameter and in the properties of its membrane, both the amplitude and the conduction velocity of the action potential will be constant, and it will behave in an all-or-none fashion. Since the amplitude of the action potential is always much greater than the threshold for stimulation, the conduction mechanism embodies a large safety factor, and the spike can be cut down a long way by changes in the conditions that adversely affect the size of the membrane potential before conduction actually fails. It will be appreciated that although there is outward current flowing through the membrane both ahead of the active region and behind it, propagation can only take place from left to right in the diagram of Figure 6.2, because the region to the rear is in a refractory state. In the living animal, action potentials normally originate at one end of a nerve, and are conducted unidirectionally away from that end. In an experimental situation where shocks are applied at the middle of an intact stretch of nerve, the membrane can of course be excited on each side of the stimulating electrode, setting up spikes travelling in both directions.

It should be clear from this description that conduction will be speeded up by an increase in the space constant for the passive spread of potential, because the resting membrane will be triggered further ahead of the advancing impulse. This is one of the reasons why large axons conduct impulses faster than small ones, for it follows from Equation (6.2) that λ is proportional to the square root of the fibre diameter. Another factor that greatly affects λ is myelinization of the nerve, and we must next discuss this in more detail.

6.2 | Saltatory conduction in myelinated nerves

In 1925, Lillie suggested that the function of the myelin sheath in vertebrate nerve fibres might be to restrict the inward and outward passage of local circuit current to the nodes of Ranvier, so causing the nerve impulse to be propagated from node to node in a series of discrete jumps. He coined the term *saltatory conduction* for this kind of process, and supported the idea with some ingenious experiments on his iron wire model. (An iron wire immersed in nitric acid of the right strength acquires a surface film along which a disturbance can be propagated by local circuit action; the mechanism has several features analogous with those of nervous conduction, for which it has served as a useful model.) The hypothesis could not be tested physiologically until methods had been developed for the dissection of isolated fibres from myelinated nerve trunks, which was first done by Kato and his school in Japan in about 1930. Ten years later Tasaki produced strong support for the saltatory theory by showing that the threshold for electrical stimulation in a single myelinated fibre was much lower at the nodes than along the internodal stretches, and that blocking by anodal polarization and by local anaesthetics was more effective at the nodes than elsewhere. In collaboration with Takeuchi, Tasaki also introduced a technique for making direct measurements of the local circuit current flowing at different positions, and this approach was subsequently perfected by Huxley and Stämpfli.

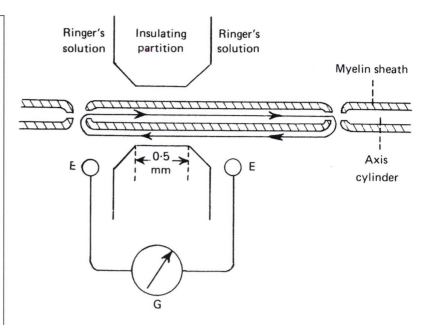

Figure 6.3 Diagram of the method used by Huxley and Stämpfli (1949) to investigate saltatory conduction in nerve. The nerve fibre is pulled through a fine hole about 40 μm in diameter in an insulator by a micromanipulator. Current flowing along the axis cylinder out of one node and into the other, as indicated by the arrows, causes a voltage drop outside the myelin sheath. The resistance of the fluid in the gap between the two pools of Ringer's solution being about half a megohm, the potential difference between them can be measured by the oscilloscope G connected to electrodes E on either side. The internodal distance in a frog's myelinated nerve fibre is about 2 mm.

The method adopted by Huxley and Stämpfli (Figure 6.3) was to pull a myelinated fibre isolated from a frog nerve through a short glass capillary mounted in a partition between two compartments filled with Ringer's solution. The fluid-filled space around the nerve inside the capillary was sufficiently narrow to have a total resistance of about 0.5 MΩ, so that the current flowing longitudinally between neighbouring nodes outside the myelin sheath gave rise to a measurable potential difference between the two sides of the partition, which could be recorded with an oscilloscope. The records of longitudinal current showed (Figure 6.4) that at all points outside any one internode the current flow was roughly the same, both in magnitude and timing. However, the peaks of current flow were displaced stepwise in time by about one tenth of a millisecond as successive nodes were traversed. In order to determine the amount of current that flowed radially into or out of the fibre, neighbouring pairs of records were subtracted from one another, since the difference between the longitudinal currents at any two points could only have arisen from current entering or leaving the axis cylinder between those points. This procedure gave the results illustrated in Figure 6.5, from which it is seen that over the internodes there was merely a slight leakage of outward current, but that at each node there was a brief pulse of outward current followed by a much larger pulse of inward current. The current flowing transversely across the myelin sheath is exactly what would be expected for a passive leak, while the restriction of inward current to the nodes proves conclusively that the sodium system operates only where the excitable membrane is accessible to the outside.

The term 'saltatory' means literally a process that is discontinuous, but it would nevertheless be wrong to suppose that only one

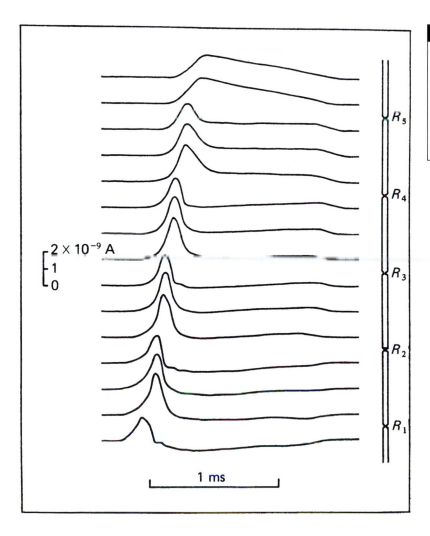

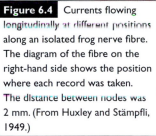

Figure 6.4 Currents flowing longitudinally at different positions along an isolated frog nerve fibre. The diagram of the fibre on the right-hand side shows the position where each record was taken. The distance between nodes was 2 mm. (From Huxley and Stämpfli, 1949.)

node is active at a time in a myelinated nerve fibre. The conduction velocity in Huxley and Stämpfli's experiments was 23 mm/ms, and the duration of the action potential was about 1.5 ms, so that the length of nerve occupied by the action potential at any moment was about 34 mm, which corresponds to a group of 17 neighbouring nodes. In the resistance network equivalent to a myelinated fibre (Figure 6.6), the values of R_n and R_i are such that the electrotonic potential would decrement passively to 0.4 between one node and the next. Since the size of the fully developed action potential is of the order of 120 mV, and since the threshold depolarization needed to excite the membrane is only about 15 mV, it again follows that the conduction mechanism works with an appreciable safety factor, and that the impulse should be able to encounter one or two inactive nodes without being blocked. Tasaki showed that two but not three nodes which had been treated with a local anaesthetic like cocaine could indeed be skipped.

Figure 6.5 Transverse currents flowing at different positions along an isolated frog nerve fibre. Each trace shows the difference between the longitudinal currents, recorded as in Figure 6.4, at the two points 0.75 mm apart indicated to the right. The vertical mark above each trace shows the time when the change in membrane potential reached its peak at that position along the fibre. Outward current is plotted upwards. (From Huxley and Stämpfli, 1949.)

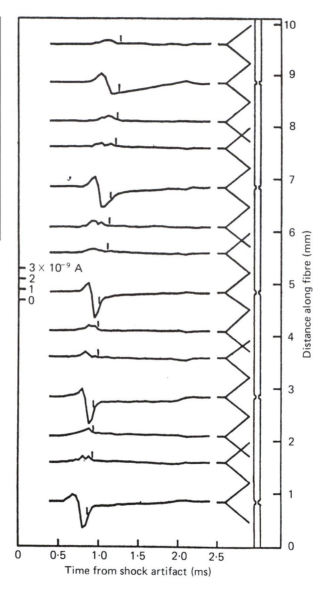

Figure 6.6 Equivalent circuit for the resistive elements of a myelinated nerve fibre. According to Tasaki (1953), for a toad fibre whose outside diameter is 12 μm and a nodal spacing 2 mm, the internal longitudinal resistance R_i is just under 20 MΩ and the resistance R_n across each node is just over 20 MΩ. In a large volume of fluid the external resistance R_o is negligibly small.

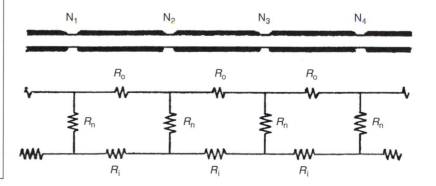

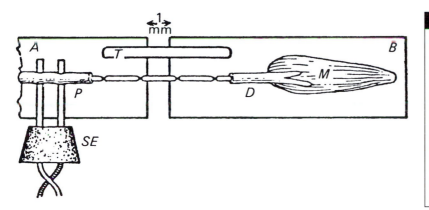

Figure 6.7 Method used by Huxley and Stämpfli (1949) to demonstrate the role of the external current pathway in a myelinated nerve fibre. A, B: insulated microscope slides; SE: stimulating electrodes; P: proximal end of frog's sciatic nerve; D: distal end of nerve; M: gastrocnemius muscle; T: moist thread providing an electrical connection between the pools of Ringer's solution on the slides.

A simple experiment which deserves mention was performed by Huxley and Stämpfli to demonstrate the importance of the external current pathway in propagation along a myelinated nerve fibre. The nerve of a frog's sciatic–gastrocnemius preparation was pared down until only one fibre was left (Figure 6.7). Stimulation of the nerve at P then caused a visible contraction of a motor unit M in the muscle. The preparation was now laid in two pools of Ringer's solution on microscope slides A and B which were electrically insulated from one another, and its position was adjusted so that part of an internode, but not a node, lay across the 1 mm air gap separating the pools. At first, stimulation at P continued to cause a muscle twitch, but soon the layer of fluid outside the myelin sheath in the air gap was dried up by evaporation, and the muscle ceased to contract. Conduction across the gap could, however, be restored by placing a wet thread T between the two pools. This demonstrated that an action potential arriving at the node just to the left of the air gap could trigger the node on the far side of the gap only when there was an electrical connection between the pools whose resistance was fairly low. On reference to Figure 6.6 it will be seen that if R_0 becomes at all large, the potential change at N_2 produced by a spike at N_1 will fall below the threshold for excitation. As has been pointed out by Tasaki, a reservation needs to be made about this experiment. Unless special precautions are taken, the stray electrical capacity between the pools may provide, for a brief pulse of current, an alternative pathway outside the dried-up myelin of the internode, whose impedance may be low enough for excitation to occur at the further node if its threshold is low. Even with such precautions, Tasaki found that impulses were still able to jump the gap if the fibre had a really low threshold, probably because simple evaporation could not make the external resistance high enough. Nevertheless, the fact that the experiment works in a clear-cut way only if the threshold is somewhat higher than it is *in vivo* does not prevent it from proving rather satisfactorily that there must be a low-impedance pathway between neighbouring nodes *outside* the myelin sheath if the nerve impulse is to be conducted along the fibre.

6.3 | Factors affecting conduction velocity

Since the passive electrotonic spread of potential along a nerve fibre is an almost instantaneous process, it may be asked why the nerve impulse is not propagated more rapidly than it actually is. In myelinated fibres the explanation is that there is a definite delay of about 0.1 ms at each node (see Figure 6.4), which represents the time necessary for Na[+] ions to move through the membrane at the node in a quantity sufficient to discharge the membrane capacity and build up a reversed potential. Conduction in a non-myelinated fibre is slower than in a myelinated fibre of the same diameter because the membrane capacity per unit length is much greater, and the delay in reversing the potential across it arises everywhere and not just at the nodes. Because the time constant for an alteration of membrane potential depends both on the magnitude of the membrane capacity and on the amount of current that flows into it, conduction velocity is affected by the values of the resistances in the equivalent electrical circuit, and also by the closeness of packing of sodium channels in the membrane, which determines the Na[+] current density. The effects of changing R_o and R_i can best be seen in isolated axons. Thus Hodgkin (1939) showed that when R_o was increased by raising an axon out of a large volume of sea water into a layer of liquid paraffin, the conduction velocity fell by about 20% in a 30 μm crab nerve fibre and by 50% in a 500 μm squid axon; and when the axon was mounted in a moist chamber lying across a series of metal bars which could be connected together by a trough of mercury, the act of short-circuiting the bars increased the velocity by 20%. More recently, del Castillo and Moore (1959) showed that a reduction in R_i brought about by inserting a silver wire down the centre of a squid axon could greatly speed up conduction.

One of the reasons why large non-myelinated fibres conduct faster than small ones is the decrease of R_i with an increase in fibre diameter. Assuming the properties of the membrane to be identical for fibres of all sizes, it can be shown that conduction velocity should be proportional to the square root of diameter. Experimentally this does not always seem to hold good, a possible explanation being that one of the ways in which giant axons are specially adapted for rapid conduction is through an increase in the number of sodium channels in the membrane. Measurements of the binding of labelled TTX have shown that the smallest fibres of all, those in garfish olfactory nerve, have the fewest channels, the site density being 35 μm[-2] as compared with 90 and 100 μm[-2] in lobster leg nerve and rabbit vagus nerve respectively (Ritchie and Rogart, 1977). However, in the squid giant axon there are about 290 TTX binding sites μm[-2] (Keynes and Ritchie, 1984). Since the flow of gating current has the consequence of increasing the effective size of the membrane capacity, there is an optimum sodium channel density above which the conduction velocity would fall off again. Hodgkin (1975) has calculated that the value found in squid is not far from the optimum.

6.4 | Factors affecting the threshold for excitation

As seen, for example, in Figure 2.7, excitation of a nerve fibre involves the rapid depolarization of the membrane to a critical level normally about 15 mV less negative than the resting potential. The critical level for excitation is the membrane potential at which the net rate of entry of Na^+ ions becomes exactly equal to the net rate of exit of K^+ ions plus a small contribution from an entry of Cl^- ions. Greater depolarization than this tips the balance in favour of Na^+, and the regenerative process described in Chapter 4 takes over and causes a rapidly accelerating inrush of Na^+. After just subthreshold depolarization, when g_{Na} will have been raised over an appreciable area of membrane, the return of the resting potential will be somewhat slow at first, and a non-propagated *local response* may be observed.

At the end of the spike the membrane is left with its Na^+ permeability mechanism inactivated and its K^+ permeability appreciably greater than normal. Both changes tend to raise the threshold for re-excitation. The partial inactivation of the Na^+ permeability system means that even to raise inward Na^+ current to the normal critical value requires more depolarization than usual, and the raised K^+ permeability means that the critical Na^+ current is actually above normal. Until the permeabilities for both ions have returned to their resting levels, and the Na^+ permeability system is fully reactivated, the shock necessary to trigger a second spike is above the normal threshold in size.

It has long been known that nerves are not readily stimulated by slowly rising currents, because they tend to *accommodate* to this type of stimulus. Accommodation arises partly because sustained depolarization brings about a long-lasting rise in K^+ permeability, and partly because at the same time it semi-permanently inactivates the Na^+ permeability mechanism. Both changes take place with an appreciable lag after the membrane potential is lowered, so that they are not effective when a constant current is first applied, but become important after a little while. They also persist for some time after the end of a stimulus, and so are responsible for the appearance of *post-cathodal depression*, which is a lowering of excitability after prolonged application of a weak cathodal current. As a result of accommodation, cathodal currents that rise more slowly than a certain limiting value do not stimulate at all, since the rise in threshold keeps pace with the depolarization.

Another familiar phenomenon is the occurrence of excitation when an anodal current is switched off. This *anode break excitation* can readily be demonstrated in isolated squid axons or frog nerves, but is not seen in freshly dissected frog muscle or in nerves stimulated *in situ* in living animals. The conditions under which anode break excitation is exhibited are that the resting potential should be well below E_K because of a steady leakage of K^+. The nerve can then be considered to be in a state of mild cathodal depression, with g_{Na} partially inactivated and g_K well above normal. The effect of anodal polarization of the membrane is to reactivate the Na^+ permeability system and to reduce the K^+ permeability, and this improved state persists for a short while after the current is switched off. While it lasts, the critical potential at which inward Na^+ current exceeds outward K^+ current may be temporarily above the membrane potential in the absence of external current. When the current is turned off, an action potential is therefore initiated.

Divalent ions like Ca^{2+} and Mg^{2+} strongly affect the threshold behaviour of excitable membranes. In squid axons, even a slight reduction in external $[Ca^{2+}]$ may set up a sinusoidal oscillation of the membrane potential, while a more drastic reduction of the Ca^{2+} will result in a spontaneous discharge of impulses at a high repetition frequency. Conversely, a rise in external $[Ca^{2+}]$ helps to stabilize the membrane and tends to raise the threshold for excitation. Changes in external $[Mg^{2+}]$ have rather similar effects on peripheral nerves, Mg^{2+} being about half as effective as Ca^{2+} in its stabilizing influence. Voltage-clamp studies by Frankenhaeuser and Hodgkin (1957) have shown that the curve relating peak Na^+ conductance to membrane potential is shifted in a positive direction along the voltage axis by raising $[Ca^{2+}]$, and is shifted in the opposite direction by lowering $[Ca^{2+}]$. However, the resting potential is rather insensitive to changes in $[Ca^{2+}]$. This readily explains the relationship between $[Ca^{2+}]$ and threshold, since a rise in $[Ca^{2+}]$ moves the critical triggering level away from the resting potential, while a fall in $[Ca^{2+}]$ moves the critical level towards it. A moderate reduction in $[Ca^{2+}]$ may bring the critical level so close to the resting potential that the membrane behaves in an unstable and oscillatory fashion, and a further reduction will then increase the amplitude of the oscillations to the point where they cause a spontaneous discharge of spikes. Although Ca^{2+} and Mg^{2+} have similar actions on the excitability of nerve and muscle fibres, they have antagonistic actions at the neuromuscular junction and at some synaptic junctions between neurons, because Ca^{2+} increases the amount of acetylcholine released by a motor nerve ending, and Mg^{2+} reduces it. Changes in the plasma calcium level in living animals may therefore give rise to tetany, but there is a complicated balance between central and peripheral effects.

6.5 | After-potentials

In many types of nerve and muscle fibre the membrane potential does not return immediately to the baseline at the foot of the action potential, but undergoes further slow variations known as after-potentials. The nomenclature of after-potentials dates from the period before the invention of intracellular recording techniques when external electrodes were used, so that an alteration of potential in the same direction as the spike itself is termed a *negative after-potential*, while a variation in the opposite direction corresponding to a hyperpolarization of the membrane is termed a *positive after-potential* (see Figure 2.3). As may be seen in Figure 2.4b, isolated squid axons display a characteristic *positive phase* which is almost completely absent in the living animals (Figure 2.4a), while frog muscle fibres have a prolonged negative after-potential (Figure 2.4h), discussed in greater detail in Section 10.2. In some mammalian nerves, both myelinated and non-myelinated, there is first a negative and then a positive after-potential. A related phenomenon, which is most marked in the smallest fibres, is the occurrence after a period of repetitive activity of a prolonged hyperpolarization of the membrane known as the post-tetanic hyperpolarization.

There is no doubt that after-potentials are always connected with changes in membrane permeability towards specific ions, but there is more than one way in which the membrane potential can be displaced either upwards or downwards. In the isolated squid axon, for example, the positive phase arises because the K^+ conductance is still relatively high at the end of the spike, whereas the Na^+ conductance is inactivated and is therefore below normal. The membrane potential consequently comes close to E_K for a short while, and then drops back as g_K and g_{Na} resume their usual resting values. The mechanism responsible for production of the positive after-potential and the post-tetanic hyperpolarization in vertebrate nerves is quite different, for it has been shown to involve an enhanced rate of extrusion of Na^+ ions by the sodium pump operating in an electrogenic mode. In other cases, a change in the relative permeability of the membrane to Cl^- and K^+ ions may play a part. There is also evidence that the presence of Schwann cells partially or wholly enveloping certain types of nerve fibre has important effects on the after-potential by slightly restricting the rate of diffusion of ions in the immediate neighbourhood of the nerve membrane.

7

Neuromuscular transmission

Skeletal muscles are innervated by motor nerves. Excitation of the motor nerve is followed by excitation and contraction of the muscle. Thus excitation of one cell, the nerve axon, produces excitation of another cell which it contacts, the muscle fibre. The region of contact between the two cells is called the *neuromuscular junction*. The process of the transmission of excitation from the nerve cell to the muscle cell is called *neuromuscular transmission*. This chapter is concerned with how this process occurs.

Regions at which transfer of electrical information between a nerve cell and another cell (which may or may not be another nerve cell) occurs are known as *synapses*, and the process of information transfer is called *synaptic transmission*. Neuromuscular transmission is just one form of synaptic transmission; we shall examine the properties of some other synapses in the following chapter.

7.1 | The neuromuscular junction

Each motor axon branches so as to supply an appreciable number of muscle fibres. Figure 7.1 shows the arrangement in most of the muscle fibres in the frog. Each axon branch loses its myelin sheath where it contracts the muscle cell and splits up into a number of fine terminals which run for a short distance along its surface. The region of the muscle fibre with which the terminals make contact is known as the *end-plate*. Structures and events occurring in the axon are called *pre-synaptic*, whereas those occurring in the muscle cell are called *post-synaptic*.

Further details of the structure in the junctional region can be determined by electron microscopy of thin sections, with the results shown in Figure 7.2. The nerve cell is separated from the muscle cell by a gap about 50 nm wide between the two apposing cell membranes. This gap is called the *synaptic cleft* and is in contact at its edges with the other extracellular spaces of the body. The axon terminal contains a large number of small membrane-bound spheres, the *synaptic vesicles*, and also a considerable number

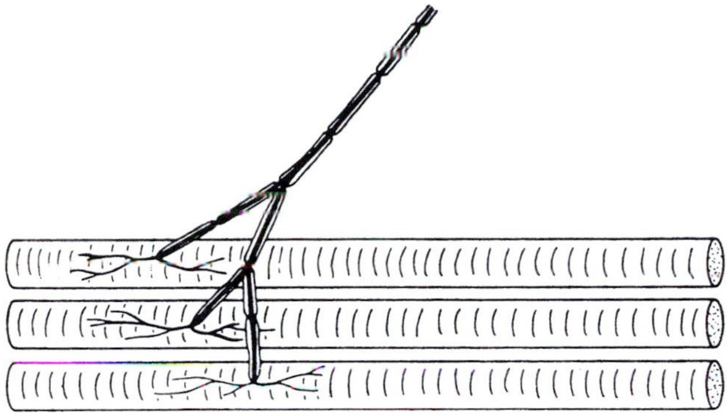

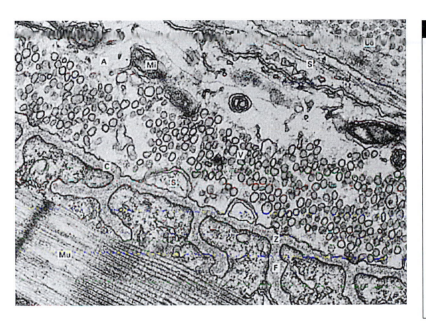

Figure 7.1 Diagrammatic picture of a vertebrate muscle motor nerve terminal. In most cases a single motor axon innervates many more muscle fibres than the three shown here.

Figure 7.2 Electron micrograph showing the structure of the frog neuromuscular junction. The axon terminal (A) runs diagonally across the middle of the section, covered by a Schwann cell (S) and collagen fibres (Co), and overlying a muscle cell (Mu). Between the axon and the muscle cell is the synaptic cleft (C). The acetylcholine receptors are concentrated at the top of a series of folds (F) in the subsynaptic membrane. The terminal contains mitochondria (Mi) and large numbers of synaptic vesicles (V). Vesicle release probably occurs at pre-synaptic active zones (Z). Magnification 27 000×. (Photograph supplied by Professor J. E. Heuser.)

of mitochondria. We shall see that the synaptic vesicles and the synaptic cleft play a vital role in the transmission process at this and other synapses.

The muscle cell membrane immediately under the axon terminal is thrown into a series of folds. The outside of the axon terminal is covered with a Schwann cell and the whole is held in position by collagen fibres.

7.2 | Chemical transmission

We must now consider the question, how does excitation in the pre-synaptic cell produce a response in the post-synaptic cell? One possibility, first suggested in the nineteenth century, is that the pre-synaptic cell might release a chemical substance which would then act as a messenger between the two cells.

An experiment to test this idea for the frog heart was carried out by O. Loewi in 1921. The heart normally beats spontaneously, but it can be inhibited by stimulation of the vagus nerve. Loewi found that the perfusion fluid from a heart which was inhibited by stimulation of the vagus would itself reduce the amplitude of the normal beat in the absence of vagal stimulation. Perfusion fluid from a heart beating normally did not have this effect. This means that stimulation of the vagus results in the release of a chemical substance, presumably from the nerve endings.

It did not take too long to show that the chemical substance was acetylcholine (Figure 8.1), a substance whose pharmacological action had previously been demonstrated by H. H. Dale. Dale and his colleagues then went on to show that acetylcholine was released from the motor nerve endings in skeletal muscle when the motor nerves were stimulated electrically.

It seems then that synaptic transmission is in most cases a chemically mediated process involving the release of a *transmitter substance* from the pre-synaptic terminals. As we shall see later, acetylcholine is an important transmitter substance, but it is not the only one.

7.3 | Post-synaptic responses

7.3.1 The end-plate potential

Stimulation of the motor nerve produces electrical responses in the muscle fibre. Our understanding of the nature of these events was greatly increased when P. Fatt and B. Katz used intracellular electrodes to study the problem in 1951. Figure 7.3 shows the experimental arrangement which they used. The glass micropipette electrode, filled with a concentrated solution of KCl, is inserted into the muscle fibre in the end-plate region. A suitable amplifier then measures the voltage between the tip of that electrode and another electrode in the external solution, so giving the electrical potential difference across the membrane. The muscle may be treated with curare (an arrow poison used by South American Indians, which

Figure 7.3 Diagram to show how the end-plate potential is recorded from a frog muscle fibre using an intracellular microelectrode.

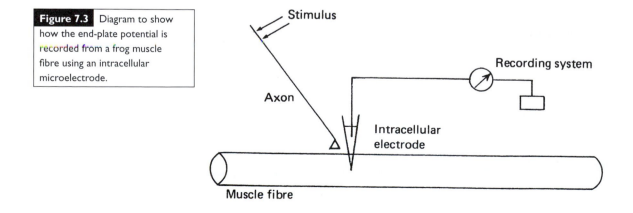

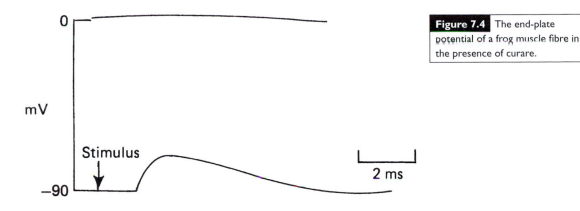

Figure 7.4 The end-plate potential of a frog muscle fibre in the presence of curare.

causes paralysis) so as to partly block the transmission process. The nerve can be stimulated via a couple of silver wire electrodes.

Figure 7.4 shows the response seen in the presence of a moderate amount of curare. There is a rapid depolarization of a few millivolts, followed by a rather slower return to the resting membrane potential. This response is not seen if the microelectrode is inserted at some distance from the end-plate, and hence it is called the *end-plate potential*. Increasing the curare concentration reduces the size of the end-plate potential.

7.3.2 Excitation of the muscle fibre

In the absence of curare the end-plate potential is its normal size, and the response recorded at the end plate is more complicated in form, as is shown in Figure 7.5*a*. The muscle cell membrane is electrically excitable so that it will carry all-or-nothing propagated action potentials, just as in the nerve axon. In the absence of curare the end-plate potential is large enough to cross the threshold for electrical excitation of the muscle cell membrane, so that an action potential arises from it and propagates along the length of the muscle fibre. The record in Figure 7.5*a* is thus a combination of end-plate potential and action potential. At some distance from the end-plate, a 'pure' action potential, free from the complicating effects of the end-plate potential, can be seen, as in Figure 7.5*b*.

The ionic basis of the muscle action potential is much the same as in the nerve axon. It is reduced in size or blocked in low sodium ion concentrations or in the presence of tetrodotoxin. So we can assume that the cell membrane contains separate channels for Na^+ and K^+ ions, both types being opened by a suitable change in membrane potential. The muscle action potential triggers the contraction of the muscle, as we shall see in Chapter 10.

7.3.3 The response to acetylcholine

We have seen that stimulation of the motor nerve causes the release of acetylcholine. Is the end-plate potential a direct result of the action of this acetylcholine on the post-synaptic membrane? Clearly a good way to test this idea is to apply acetylcholine to the post-synaptic

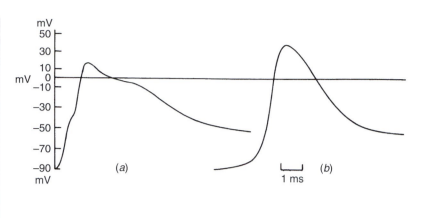

Figure 7.5 Action potentials produced in a frog muscle fibre by stimulation of its motor nerve axon. In trace (*a*) the microelectrode was positioned at the end-plate region, so that the response includes an end-plate potential plus the action potential which it gives rise to. In trace (*b*) the microelectrode was positioned at some distance from the end-plate so that no end-plate potential component is recorded. (Based on Fatt and Katz, 1951.)

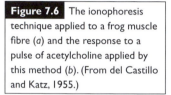
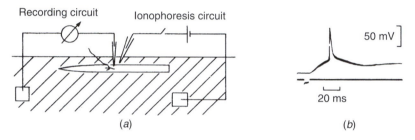

Figure 7.6 The ionophoresis technique applied to a frog muscle fibre (*a*) and the response to a pulse of acetylcholine applied by this method (*b*). (From del Castillo and Katz, 1955.)

membrane and see if it produces a depolarization. If it does not, we shall have to think again, but if it does, then the idea becomes much better established as a result of passing this test.

The best way of applying acetylcholine to the post-synaptic membrane is by means of a technique known as ionophoresis or iontophoresis. Acetylcholine is a positively charged ion (Figure 8.1), and so it will move in an electric field. Hence it can be ejected from a small pipette by passing current through the pipette, as is shown in Figure 7.6. Thus a brief, highly localized 'pulse' of acetylcholine can be applied to the post-synaptic membrane. Such a pulse produces a depolarization of the muscle fibre which is very similar to the end-plate potential (Figure 7.6*b*). The pharmacological properties of the response are also similar to those of the end-plate potential; it is reduced in the presence of curare, for example. So it seems very reasonable to conclude that the end-plate potential is indeed produced by the acetylcholine which is released from the motor nerve ending.

7.3.4 Ionic current flow during the end-plate potential

Fatt and Katz suggested that the end-plate potential was produced by a general increase in the ionic permeability of the post-synaptic membrane. A closer look at the problem was provided by A. and N. Takeuchi, who used a voltage-clamp technique on frog muscle fibres to examine the post-synaptic current flow during the response to a

(a)

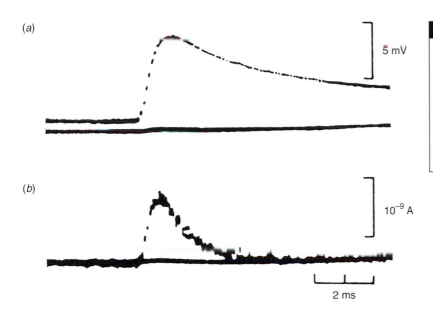

5 mV

(b)

10^{-9} A

2 ms

Figure 7.7 Measurement of the end-plate potential and end-plate current in a curarized frog muscle fibre. Trace (a) shows the EPP, recorded in the usual manner. Trace (b) shows the EPC recorded from the same end-plate with the membrane potential clamped at its resting level. (From Takeuchi and Takeuchi, 1959.)

nerve impulse. They found that the duration of the end-plate current flow is briefer than the end-plate potential, as is shown in Figure 7.7. This is because the 'tail' of the end-plate potential is caused by a re-charging of the membrane capacitance, which does not occur when the membrane potential is clamped.

The membrane potential can be clamped at different values. When this is done it is found that the amplitude of the end-plate cur-rent varies linearly with membrane potential (Figure 7.8). This linear relation between current and voltage is just what we would expect from Ohm's law: it indicates that the conductance of the membrane at the peak of the end-plate current is constant and not affected by the membrane potential. This is in marked contrast to the situation in the nerve axon, where the Na^+ and K^+ permeabilities of the mem-brane are most strongly altered by changes in membrane potential.

The point at which the line through the experimental points in Figure 7.8 crosses the voltage axis is called the *reversal potential*. If the membrane potential is made more positive than this we would expect the end-plate current to flow in the opposite direction, as indeed it does.

The reversal potential is the membrane potential at which the net ionic current is zero. If only one type of ion were flowing, the reversal potential would be at the equilibrium potential for that ion; for example, it would be about +50 mV if only sodium ions were flowing. But if more than one type of ion flows during the end-plate current, then the reversal potential will be somewhere between the various equilibrium potentials for the different ions. The actual reversal potential, at about −15 mV in the Takeuchis' experiments, is compatible with the idea that both Na^+ and K^+ ions flow during the end-plate current. If we alter the equilibrium potential for one of the ions involved, then the reversal potential will also alter. The

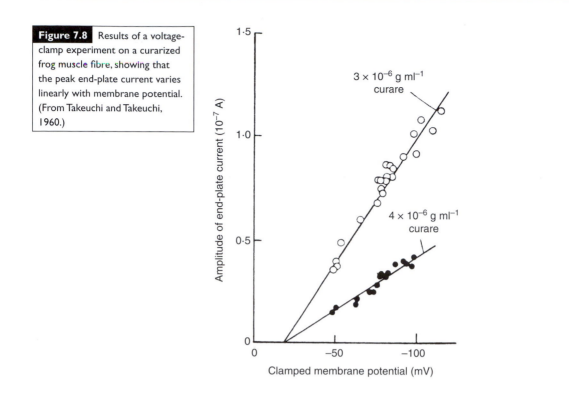

Figure 7.8 Results of a voltage-clamp experiment on a curarized frog muscle fibre, showing that the peak end-plate current varies linearly with membrane potential. (From Takeuchi and Takeuchi, 1960.)

Takeuchis did just this by changing the ionic concentrations in the external solutions. They found that alterations in Na⁺ and K⁺ ion concentrations both altered the reversal potential, whereas alterations in Cl⁻ ion concentration did not. This means that the end-plate current consists of a flow of Na⁺ and K⁺ ions. To put it another way, acetylcholine increases the permeability of the post-synaptic membrane to both Na⁺ and K⁺ ions simultaneously.

7.3.5 Acetylcholine receptors and single-channel responses

It is now generally accepted that most pharmacological agents act at specific molecular sites on the cell membrane, called *receptors*. Only cells which possess the appropriate receptor will respond to a particular agent. In accordance with this view, we would expect to find specific acetylcholine receptors on the post-synaptic membrane at the neuromuscular junction.

The substance α-bungarotoxin, a polypeptide found in the venom of a Formosan snake, causes neuromuscular block by binding tightly to the acetylcholine receptors. Using radioactive toxin (made by acetylating the toxin with ³H-acetic anhydride) it is a simple matter to show by autoradiography that the toxin rapidly becomes attached to the post-synaptic membrane at the end-plate regions. By counting the grains of silver produced in the autoradiograph, it is then possible to count the number of toxin molecules that have been bound and from this to estimate the number of receptors present.

The results suggest that there are about 3×10^7 binding sites per end-plate in mammals, corresponding to an average density in the region of 10^4 sites per μm^2.

Since combination of acetylcholine with the receptors causes an increase in membrane permeability to Na^+ and K^+ ions, it seems very likely that each receptor is closely associated with an *ion channel* through which this ionic flow can occur. It would normally be closed and would open for a short time when acetylcholine combines with the receptor.

Direct evidence for this view was provided in experiments by E. Neher and B. Sakmann, for which they developed the patch-clamp technique (see Figure 4.17). They used frog muscle fibres whose motor nerve supply had been cut some time previously. Following this procedure the whole surface of the fibre becomes sensitive to acetylcholine and contains a low density of acetylcholine receptors. The polished tip of a microelectrode can then be pushed against the fibre membrane, so that the current flow through a small patch of membrane containing only a few receptors can be measured.

Neher and Sakmann found that, when the patch electrode contains acetylcholine, individual channels each produce a square pulse of current lasting up to a few milliseconds. The durations of successive current pulses were variable, but their amplitudes were constant, as is shown in Figure 7.9. This suggests that the channel is either open or shut, and that it can only open when it combines with acetylcholine. Probably two molecules of acetylcholine need to combine with each receptor in order to open the channel. The end-plate potential is thus produced when a large number of channels open more or less at the same time.

7.3.6 The molecular structure of the acetylcholine receptor

The electric organs of the electric ray *Torpedo* provide a rich source of acetylcholine receptors. They can be isolated by using their specific binding to the snake venom α-bungarotoxin. The receptors are pentameric proteins with a total molecular weight of about 290 kDa.

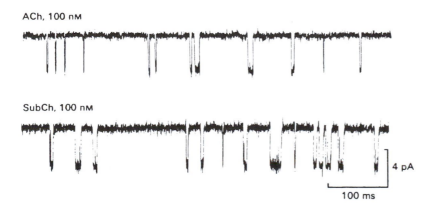

ACh, 100 nm

SubCh, 100 nm

4 pA

100 ms

Figure 7.9 Patch-clamp records of single-channel currents from frog end-plates. The upper record shows the response to acetylcholine, the lower one shows the response to suberyldicholine. (From Colquhoun and Sakmann, 1985.)

The subunits are called the α, β, γ and δ chains; there are two α chains in each receptor and one of each of the others. The binding sites for acetylcholine are located on the α chains.

The acetylcholine receptor was the first ion channel to be sequenced by using recombinant DNA techniques. In 1982 the Kyoto University group (Noda and his colleagues) published the amino-acid sequence of the α subunit, and sequences for the other subunits soon followed. The subunits varied in size from 437 amino acids (50 kDa) for the α chain to 501 amino acids (58 kDa) for the δ chain.

The sequences for the four subunits show considerable homology. They all have four hydrophobic segments which probably form membrane-crossing helices (Figure 7.10a, b). The long section from the beginning of the chain to the first membrane-crossing helix is apparently all on the outside of the membrane. It contains disulfide crosslinks and sites for the attachment of sugars. In the α chain it contains the sites for binding acetylcholine and α-bungarotoxin.

How are the five subunits put together to form the whole complex? N. Unwin has used a sophisticated technique known as cryo-electron microscopy to answer this question. Nicotinic acetylcholine receptors can be isolated from *Torpedo* electric organ as regular close-packed arrays in tubular form. These arrays can be frozen and examined in the electron microscope, and the images subjected to Fourier analysis to give a three-dimensional map of the electron density in the molecule. Unwin was also able to examine the effects of acetylcholine on the structure by spraying it at the receptors just milliseconds before freezing them in liquid ethane at −178 °C.

The results of this procedure show that the five subunits form a receptor that has a large extracellular component to accommodate the two acetylcholine binding sites on the α subunits. The wide vestibule in the extracellular region narrows to a fine pore in the transmembrane region. At this narrow region the pore is lined by dense bent rods, which are probably the M2 segments of the five subunits. Figure 7.10b gives an impression of the whole structure.

Figure 7.10 Diagrams of the molecular structure of the nicotinic acetylcholine receptor/channel. The complex consists of five subunits (a); the two α-subunits contain acetylcholine binding sites. The amino acid chain of each subunit contains four membrane-crossing segments (b).

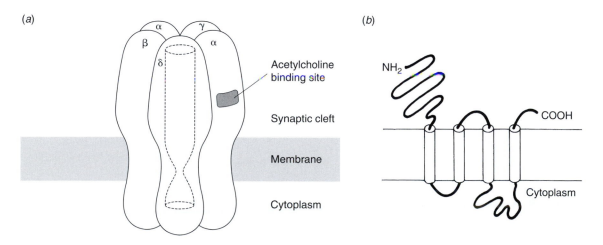

In the resting state Unwin's model suggests that the channel is closed at its narrowest part by a large hydrophobic leucine residue. When acetylcholine binds to the α-subunits, the M2 segments rotate somewhat to move these leucine residues out of the way so that cations can flow through the channel pore.

It is instructive to compare the nicotinic acetylcholine receptor channel with the voltage-gated channels described in Chapter 5. Unlike them, it is not gated by a change in membrane potential, and so, not surprisingly, there are no voltage sensors corresponding to the S4 segments of the voltage-gated channels. It belongs to a group of *neurotransmitter-gated channels*, which are themselves part of the general class of *ligand-gated channels*, which open when they bind a particular ligand molecule.

How can we be sure that the four subunits are sufficient to produce a functional receptor? The oocytes of the African clawed toad *Xenopus* have provided a most useful method for solving this problem.

Oocytes are large cells which are about to develop into mature eggs. They possess the normal translation machinery and so they will respond to the injection of messenger RNA by making the protein for which it codes. Barnard and his colleagues injected oocytes with messenger RNA from *Torpedo* electric organ; two days later the oocyte would respond to application of acetylcholine by ionophoresis with a rapid depolarization, as is shown in Figure 7.11.

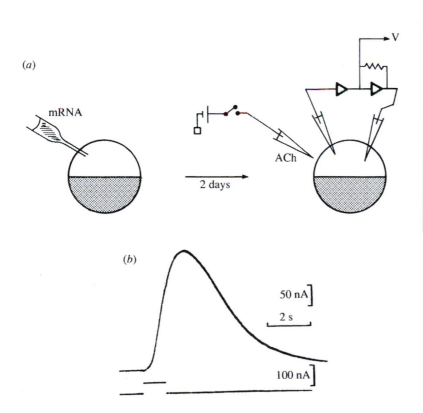

Figure 7.11 Expression of acetylcholine receptors in *Xenopus* oocytes. Messenger RNA from *Torpedo* electric organ is injected into an oocyte; two days later the oocyte membrane potential is voltage-clamped while acetylcholine is applied by ionophoresis (*a*). The record (*b*) shows the current response (upper trace) to acetylcholine; the lower trace monitors the ionophoresis current. (From Barnard et al., 1982.)

Molecular-cloning methods can be used to make messenger RNA coding for the different subunits of the acetylcholine receptor. Only when messenger RNAs for all four of the subunits were injected would the oocyte respond to application of acetylcholine. This shows that all four of the subunits are necessary for production of a functional receptor. It also shows that no extra components are required, so providing excellent confirmation for the conclusions of the recombinant DNA work.

Substances other than acetylcholine can combine with the receptors. Blocking agents such as α-bungarotoxin and curare combine with the receptors without opening their channels. Curare and some other compounds of this type are useful as muscular relaxing agents in surgery. Agonists of acetylcholine, such as nicotine and carbachol, combine with the receptors and do open the channels, so they induce ionic flow just as acetylcholine does.

In the disease myasthenia gravis it seems likely that the body produces antibodies to the neuromuscular acetylcholine receptor, resulting in partial neuromuscular block.

7.3.7   Acetylcholinesterase

The enzyme acetylcholinesterase hydrolyses acetylcholine to form choline and acetic acid. Histochemical staining shows that this enzyme is greatly concentrated in the synaptic cleft and especially in the folds of the subsynaptic membrane. Its function is to hydrolyse the acetylcholine so as to limit the time during which it is active after being released by a motor nerve impulse.

A number of substances inhibit the action of acetylcholinesterase; they are known as *anticholinesterases*. They include the alkaloid eserine and the organophosphorus insecticides.

7.4 | Pre-synaptic events

The pre-synaptic nerve terminal is much smaller than the post-synaptic muscle fibre, and so it is much more difficult to investigate its properties directly. It is not possible, for example, to insert an intracellular microelectrode into it. Fortunately, however, the main feature of interest to us is the release of acetylcholine, and we can measure this relatively easily by recording the responses of the post-synaptic cell.

7.4.1   The quantal release of acetylcholine

In the resting muscle small fluctuations in membrane potential occur at the end-plate region (Figure 7.12). They follow much the same time course as do end-plate potentials, but are only about 0.5 mV in size, hence they are called *miniature end-plate potentials*. They are reduced in size by curare and increased in size by anticholinesterases, and so it looks as though they are produced by the spontaneous release of 'packets' of acetylcholine from the motor

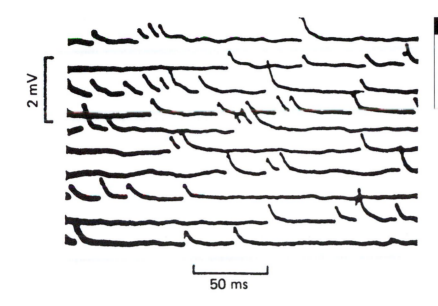

Figure 7.12 A series of membrane potential records from a frog neuromuscular junction showing miniature end-plate potentials. (From Fatt and Katz, 1952.)

2 mV

50 ms

nerve ending. Kuffler and Yoshikami compared their size with those of responses to ionophoretic application of acetylcholine; they concluded that each miniature end-plate potential is produced by the action of just under 10 000 molecules of acetylcholine.

An excess of Mg^{2+} ions blocks neuromuscular transmission by reducing the amount of acetylcholine released per nerve impulse. Del Castillo and Katz found that the size of the small end-plate potentials produced under these conditions fluctuates in a stepwise manner. Each step was about the size of a miniature end-plate potential. They therefore suggested that acetylcholine is released from the motor nerve terminals in discrete 'packets' or *quanta*. The normal end-plate potential is then the response to some hundreds of these quanta, all released at the same time following the arrival of a nerve impulse at the axon terminal. Miniature end-plate potentials are the result of spontaneous release of single quanta.

But why should acetylcholine be discharged from nerve endings in packets of nearly 10 000 molecules? The axon terminals contain large numbers of *synaptic vesicles* about 50 nm in diameter (Figure 7.2). Similar vesicles have been found in the pre-synaptic terminals at other synapses where chemical transmission occurs. Del Castillo and Katz suggested that they contain the chemical transmitter substance (acetylcholine at the neuromuscular junction), and that the discharge of the contents of one vesicle into the synaptic cleft corresponds to the release of one quantum of the transmitter.

Confirmation of this idea has since been provided by biochemical separation techniques, especially by Whittaker and his colleagues. A tissue containing a large number of nerve endings (such as brain tissue or electric organ) is first homogenized and then centrifuged. Nearly pure fractions of synaptic vesicles have been obtained from electric organs by this method, and it is found that they contain acetylcholine. They also contain some adenosine triphosphate (ATP), but the function of this is not clear.

7.4.2   Depolarization and calcium entry

The normal trigger for the release of acetylcholine is the arrival of a nerve action potential at the terminal. Katz and Miledi found that, if the action potential is blocked by tetrodotoxin, acetylcholine can still be released by depolarizing the terminal with applied current. However, this current is only effective when Ca^{2+} ions are present in the external solution. Axon terminals contain numbers of voltage-gated calcium channels. It seems probable that these open during the action potential so that Ca^{2+} ions enter the terminal and act as a trigger for the release of the contents of the vesicles.

7.4.3   Synaptic delay

There is a short delay between the arrival of an action potential in the terminal and the ensuing depolarization of the muscle cell. In frog muscle at 17 °C, the minimum time is about 0.5 ms. The major part of this delay is probably taken up by the processes involving Ca^{2+} ions in the pre-synaptic terminal. In addition the acetylcholine takes a little time to diffuse across the synaptic cleft and to combine with the acetylcholine receptors to open the ionic channels.

7.4.4   Facilitation and depression

When the motor axon is stimulated repetitively, the successful end-plate potentials produced are often of different sizes. At the beginning of a series, and especially in low Ca^{2+} ion concentrations, successive potentials increase in size. This phenomenon is known as *facilitation*. The larger responses are made up of more quantal units. Thus facilitation seems to be caused by an enhancement of the release process, perhaps because of an accumulation of Ca^{2+} ions at some site within the pre-synaptic terminal.

The opposite of facilitation is *depression*, in which succeeding responses are smaller and composed of fewer quantal units. Depression occurs when a large number of quanta have recently been released, as in the later stages of a train of stimuli in the presence of an adequate concentration of Ca^{2+} ions. It appears to be caused by a temporary reduction in the number of vesicles which are available for release.

Synaptic transmission in the nervous system

The functioning of the nervous system depends largely on the interactions between its constituent nerve cells, and these interactions take place at synapses. In most cases synaptic transmission is chemical in nature, so that, as in neuromuscular transmission, the pre-synaptic cell releases a chemical transmitter substance which produces a response in the post-synaptic cell. There are a few examples of electrically transmitting synapses, which we shall consider briefly at the end of this chapter.

Acetylcholine is only one of a range of different neurotransmitters. Figure 8.1 shows some of the variety found in the central nervous system. For a long time it was thought that any one cell would only release one neurotransmitter, but several cases where two of them are released at the same time are now known.

Different chemically transmitting synapses differ in the details of their anatomy, but some features are common to all of them. In the pre-synaptic terminal the transmitter substance is packaged in synaptic vesicles. The pre- and post-synaptic cells are separated by a synaptic cleft into which the contents of the vesicles are discharged. There are specific receptors for the neurotransmitter on the post-synaptic membrane.

Just as with the neuromuscular junction, our knowledge of how synapses work was greatly affected by the invention of the intracellular microelectrode. Much of the fundamental work with this technique was performed by J. C. Eccles and his colleagues on the spinal motoneurons of the cat, so it is with these that we shall begin our account of synapses between neurons.

8.1 | Synaptic excitation in motoneurons

Motoneurons are the nerve cells which directly innervate skeletal muscle fibres. Their cell bodies lie in the ventral horn of the spinal cord, and their axons pass out to the peripheral nerves via the ventral roots. The cell body, or soma, is about 70 μm across, and extends into a number of fine branching processes, the dendrites, which

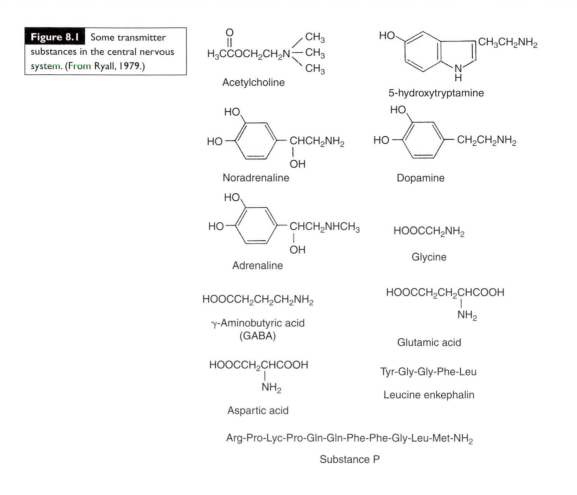

Figure 8.1 Some transmitter substances in the central nervous system. (From Ryall, 1979.)

Acetylcholine

5-hydroxytryptamine

Noradrenaline

Dopamine

Adrenaline

Glycine

γ-Aminobutyric acid (GABA)

Glutamic acid

Aspartic acid

Tyr-Gly-Gly-Phe-Leu

Leucine enkephalin

Arg-Pro-Lyc-Pro-Gln-Gln-Phe-Phe-Gly-Leu-Met-NH$_2$

Substance P

may be up to 1 mm long. The surface of the soma and dendrites is covered with small pre-synaptic nerve terminals, and these regions of contact show the typical features of chemically transmitting synapses: a synaptic cleft and synaptic vesicles in the pre-synaptic cell.

Intracellular recording shows that motoneurons have a resting potential of about −70 mV. Depolarization of the membrane by about 10 mV results in the production of an action potential which propagates along the axon to the nerve terminals. Experiments involving the injection of various ions into motoneurons indicate that the ionic basis of their resting and action potentials is much the same as in squid axons. That is to say, the resting potential is slightly less than the K$^+$ equilibrium potential, the action potential is caused primarily by a regenerative increase in Na$^+$ permeability, and the ionic gradients necessary for these potentials are dependent upon an active extrusion of Na$^+$ ions.

8.1.1   Excitatory post-synaptic potentials

Some of the pre-synaptic terminals on any particular motoneuron are the endings of sensory axons (known as group Ia fibres) from muscle spindles in the muscle which the motoneuron innervates.

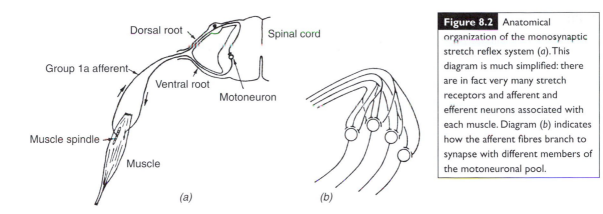

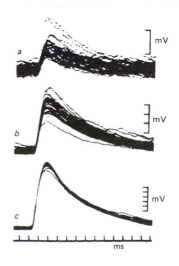

Figure 8.2 Anatomical organization of the monosynaptic stretch reflex system (*a*). This diagram is much simplified: there are in fact very many stretch receptors and afferent and efferent neurons associated with each muscle. Diagram (*b*) indicates how the afferent fibres branch to synapse with different members of the motoneuronal pool.

Stretching the muscle excites these axons, which may then excite the motoneurons supplying the muscle so that it contracts. This system is known as a monosynaptic reflex (Figure 8.2). The knee-jerk reflex is a familiar example.

The post-synaptic responses of motoneurons can be observed by means of a microelectrode inserted into the soma. Stimulation of the group Ia fibres which synapse with a particular motoneuron produces brief depolarizations, as is shown in Figure 8.3. These responses are called *excitatory post-synaptic potentials* or EPSPs. Their form is similar to that of the end-plate potential in a curarized skeletal muscle fibre: there is a fairly rapid rising phase followed by a slower return to the resting potential.

Each EPSP is the result of action potentials in a number of presynaptic fibres. With low intensity stimulation applied to the nerve from the muscle, only a few of the group Ia fibres are excited and the EPSP is correspondingly small. As we increase the stimulus intensity, more and more of the group Ia fibres are excited and the EPSP correspondingly grows in size. Thus the responses produced by activity at different synapses on the same motoneuron can add together. This phenomenon is known as *spatial summation*. If a second EPSP is elicited before the first one has died away, the net depolarization will be enhanced as the second EPSP adds to the first. This is known as *temporal summation*.

A large EPSP will be sufficient to cross the threshold for production of an action potential. This then propagates along the axon out to the periphery, where it ultimately produces contraction of the muscle fibres innervated by the axon.

The membrane potential of a motoneuron can be altered by inserting a special double-barrelled microelectrode into it and passing current down one barrel while the other is used to record the membrane potential. When the membrane potential is progressively depolarized, the EPSP decreases in size and eventually becomes reversed in sign. The reversal potential is about 0 mV. This suggests that the EPSP is produced by a change in ionic conductance which is

Figure 8.3 Excitatory post-synaptic potentials (EPSPs) recorded from a cat spinal motoneuron in response to stimuli of increasing intensity (from *a* to *c*) applied to the group Ia afferent fibres from the muscle. (From Coombs *et al.*, 1955a.)

independent of membrane potential, just as is the end-plate potential in muscle. The ions involved are probably Na⁺ and K⁺, just as they are in the end-plate potential.

These similarities between the EPSP and the end-plate potential, together with the existence of synaptic vesicles in the pre-synaptic terminals, suggest that the EPSP is produced by a neurotransmitter released from the group Ia terminals. There is good evidence, especially from spinal neurons grown in cell culture, that the transmitter is glutamate and that it acts by binding to glutamate receptors on the post-synaptic membrane. These receptors act as ion channels that open when the receptor binds glutamate.

Glutamate receptors have been cloned so that some deductions can be made about their structure. The subunits have three membrane-crossing segments and one (M2) that dips into and out of the membrane from the cytoplasmic side. This is rather different from the situation in the nicotinic acetylcholine receptor, and indeed there is no homology between the amino-acid sequences of the two receptors. A whole channel is made up of four or perhaps five subunits, presumably surrounding a central pore.

8.2 | Inhibition in motoneurons

If the contraction of a particular limb muscle is to be effective in producing movement, it is essential that the muscles which oppose this action (the antagonists) should be relaxed. In the monosynaptic stretch reflex this is brought about by *inhibition* of the motoneurons of the antagonistic muscles. Figure 8.4 shows the arrangement of the neurons involved. We have seen that group Ia fibres from the stretch receptors in a particular muscle synapse with motoneurons innervating that muscle. They also synapse with small interneurons which themselves innervate the

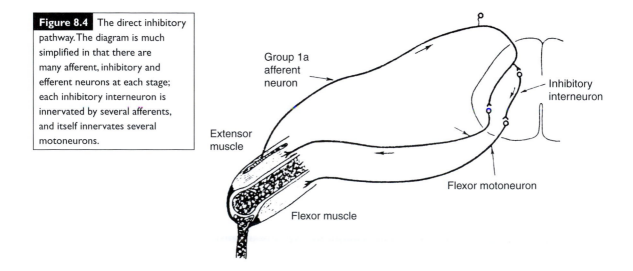

Figure 8.4 The direct inhibitory pathway. The diagram is much simplified in that there are many afferent, inhibitory and efferent neurons at each stage; each inhibitory interneuron is innervated by several afferents, and itself innervates several motoneurons.

Group 1a afferent neuron

Inhibitory interneuron

Extensor muscle

Flexor motoneuron

Flexor muscle

motoneurons of antagonistic muscles. It is these interneurons which exert the inhibitory action on the motoneurons.

This inhibitory action can be examined by inserting a microelectrode into a motoneuron and stimulating the group Ia fibres from an antagonistic muscle. Figure 8.5 shows the results of such an experiment. The responses consist of small hyperpolarizing potentials known as *inhibitory post-synaptic potentials*, or IPSPs.

The form of the IPSP is very similar to that of the EPSP, apart from the fact that it is normally hyperpolarizing. Displacement of the motoneuron membrane potential produces more or less linear changes in the size of the IPSP, with a reversal potential at about -80 mV. This is near to the equilibrium potentials of both Cl^- and K^+ ions. Injection of Cl^- ions into the soma causes an immediate reduction in the reversal potential, so that the IPSP becomes a depolarizing response at the normal membrane potential. This suggests very strongly that an increase in the Cl^- ion conductance of the post-synaptic membrane is involved in the production of the IPSP.

We can conclude that the IPSP in a spinal motoneuron is produced in a way very similar to that of the EPSP and the end-plate potential. An action potential arriving at the pre-synaptic terminal causes release of the transmitter substance (glycine in this case) into the synaptic cleft. The glycine combines with glycine receptors which act as ion channels whose opening allows Cl^- ions to flow into the post-synaptic cell, so producing the IPSP.

In the brain most of the inhibitory responses are produced not by glycine, but by gamma-aminobutyric acid (GABA). GABA receptors are of two types: the $GABA_A$ receptors can act as ion channels, whereas the $GABA_B$ receptors do not. The structure and properties of the $GABA_A$ receptors are very similar to those of glycine receptors.

The subunits of the $GABA_A$ and glycine receptors have very similar sequences, and show some identity with those of the nicotinic acetylcholine receptor; the three receptors form a gene family with, we presume, a common evolutionary origin. It is likely that each receptor consists of five subunits surrounding a central pore, just as in the nicotinic acetylcholine receptor.

IPSPs show spatial and temporal summation just as EPSPs do.

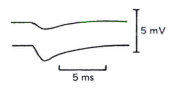

Figure 8.5 Inhibitory post-synaptic potentials (IPSPs) in a cat spinal motoneuron, produced by stimulating the group Ia fibres from the antagonistic muscle. The stimulus intensity was higher for the lower trace than for the upper, so that more group Ia fibres were excited. (From Coombs *et al.*, 1955b.)

8.3 | Interaction of IPSPs with EPSPs

The peak depolarization during an EPSP is reduced if there is an overlap in time with an IPSP. If the EPSP was just large enough to elicit an action potential in the absence of the IPSP, then the IPSP may reduce the EPSP so that it no longer crosses the threshold for production of an action potential (Figure 8.6). When the motoneuron is prevented from producing an action potential in this way it cannot induce muscular contraction and so it is effectively inhibited.

The motoneuron is in a sense a decision-making device. The decision to be made is whether or not to 'fire', that is to say whether

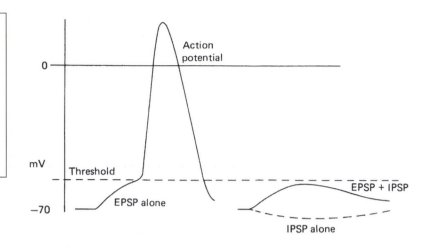

Figure 8.6 Interaction between excitatory and inhibitory PSPs in the motoneuron. The diagram shows an EPSP which is just large enough to cross the threshold for excitation of an action potential. When an IPSP occurs at the same time, the combined result is insufficient to cause excitation, and so no action potential is propagated out along the axon.

or not to send an action potential out along the axon towards the muscle. If the incoming excitatory synaptic action is sufficiently in excess of the incoming inhibitory action, the resulting depolarization will cross the threshold for production of an action potential and the motoneuron will 'fire'. But a reduction in synaptic excitation or an increase in synaptic inhibition will make the membrane potential more negative so that it drops below the threshold and the motoneuron ceases firing. We should remember that the motoneuron receives excitatory and inhibitory inputs from many sources, so that, for example, a 'decision' based on inhibition from group Ia fibres from an antagonistic muscle may be 'over-ruled' by excitatory inputs for neurons descending from the brain.

8.4 | Pre-synaptic inhibition

The inhibitory process described so far involves the production of hyperpolarizing responses in the post-synaptic cell, and it is thus known as post-synaptic inhibition. Most inhibitory interactions between nerve cells are of this type. In some cases, however, inhibition occurs without there being any post-synaptic response to the inhibitory input alone (Figure 8.7). This is thought to be caused by synaptic inputs to the pre-synaptic terminal, which reduce the size of the pre-synaptic action potential and so reduce the number of transmitter quanta released. Electron microscopy shows the presence of *serial synapses* (Figure 8.7c), in good agreement with this view. The process is known as pre-synaptic inhibition.

8.5 | Slow synaptic potentials

Dale used pharmacological criteria to distinguish two types of response to acetylcholine in peripheral tissues. *Nicotinic* responses are mimicked by nicotine and blocked by curare, whereas *muscarinic* responses are mimicked by muscarine and blocked by atropine. Correspondingly, we find there are two distinct types of acetylcholine receptor, nicotinic and muscarinic. Nicotinic receptors occur at the skeletal neuromuscular junction, muscarinic receptors mediate the responses of heart muscle to vagal stimulation. Both types are found in sympathetic ganglia, where they produce different types of responses: let us have a look at them.

The post-synaptic cells in bullfrog sympathetic ganglia show a number of different types of synaptic activity, as is shown in Figure 8.8. A single stimulus to the pre-ganglionic fibres produces a fast EPSP which may be large enough to produce an action potential in the post-ganglionic fibres. The response is blocked by curare and can be mimicked by acetylcholine. Thus the mechanism of production of the fast EPSP is similar to that at the neuromuscular junction: it is mediated by nicotinic acetylcholine receptors in which a cation-selective channel opens when acetylcholine is bound to it.

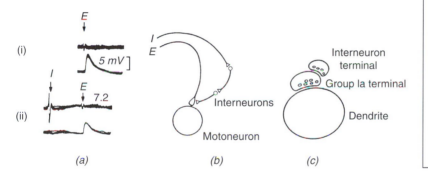

(a)

(b)

(c)

Figure 8.7 Pre-synaptic inhibition. (a) (i) shows the EPSP produced in a motoneuron in response to stimulation (at time E) of the group Ia fibres innervating it. When a suitable inhibitory nerve is stimulated just beforehand (at I), the EPSP is reduced in size although there is no IPSP or other post-synaptic event associated with the inhibitory stimulation, as is shown in (a) (ii). (b) shows the probable nervous pathways and (c) shows the serial synapses which are thought to be involved. ((a) from Eccles, 1964.)

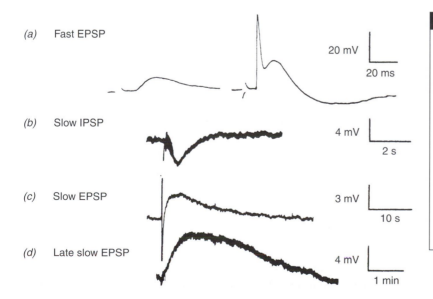

(a) Fast EPSP

(b) Slow IPSP

(c) Slow EPSP

(d) Late slow EPSP

Figure 8.8 Fast and slow synaptic responses in a frog sympathetic ganglion neuron. The trace on the left in (a) shows the fast EPSP produced by a single pre-ganglionic stimulus; a stronger stimulus (right) excites more pre-ganglionic fibres giving a larger EPSP which is sufficient to produce an action potential. In (b) to (d) the fast EPSP is blocked by a curare-like compound; repetitive stimulation at various sites then produces three different types of slow response. Note the different time scales. (From Kuffler, 1980.)

In some cells a slow EPSP with a much longer time course occurs after the fast EPSP. Similar responses are seen after application of acetylcholine. The slow EPSP is unaffected by curare, but is blocked by atropine, hence the receptors which mediate it are muscarinic. Conductance measurements show that the slow EPSP is produced by the closure of ion channels selective for K^+ ions.

In other cells the fast nicotinic EPSP is followed by a slow, hyper-polarizing IPSP. This also is muscarinic, and probably involves the opening of potassium channels. Finally, a long period of repetitive stimulation of the pre-ganglionic fibres produces a depolarization which lasts for a few minutes; it is called the late slow EPSP. The neurotransmitter which produces this is a peptide similar in structure to the luteinizing-hormone releasing hormone.

Slow potentials are widely distributed. Their time course and their long latency could be explained if channel opening or closing is mediated by an indirect process involving intermediate steps between binding at the receptor and the response of the channel, rather than the direct link which occurs in fast-acting receptors acting as ion channels. The intermediate steps involve the activation of G proteins and often the production of intracellular 'second messengers'.

The second messenger concept was first introduced to describe the role of cyclic 3´,5´-adenosine monophosphate (cyclic AMP) in hormone action. Combination of a hormone with its receptor activates a G protein (so called because it needs to bind guanosine triphosphate to become active) which in turn activates the enzyme adenylate cyclase. This produces cyclic AMP which then alters the physiological properties of the cell in some way, such as by opening or closing ion channels. Neurotransmitters may act in a similar fashion, or may utilise a different second messenger such as inositol *tris*phosphate. In some cases the G protein may act directly on the membrane channel without producing a second messenger. Figure 8.9 summarizes the various ways in which neurotransmitters may affect channels, and Table 8.1 outlines some of the various neurotransmitter receptors.

8.6 | G-protein-linked receptors

The best known of the neurotransmitter receptors that act via G proteins are the muscarinic acetylcholine receptor and the β-adrenergic receptor. There are a number of subtypes of each of these, as is indicated in Table 8.1. β-adrenergic receptors mediate many of the responses to noradrenaline in smooth and heart muscle cells, as we shall see in Chapters 12 and 13.

Molecular cloning techniques show that the muscarinic acetylcholine receptor and the β-adrenergic receptor (Figure 8.10) are strikingly similar in structure, with identical amino acids at 30% of their residues. Their amino-acid sequences are also surprisingly similar to that of the visual pigment rhodopsin, with 23% homology in each case. All three molecules have seven hydrophobic membrane-crossing

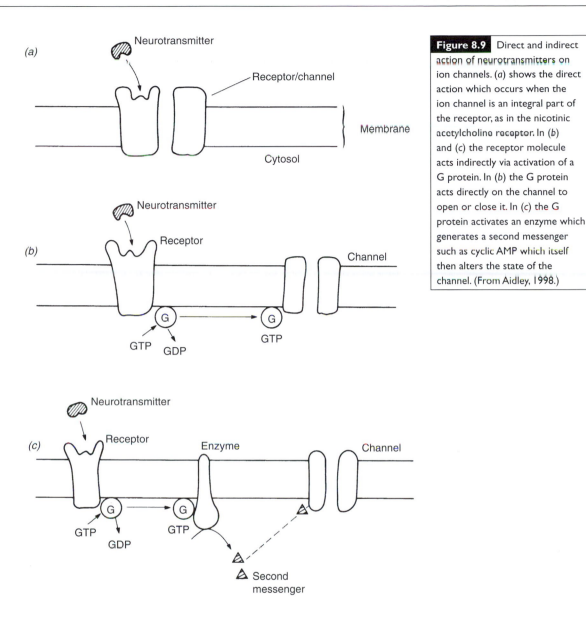

Figure 8.9 Direct and indirect action of neurotransmitters on ion channels. (a) shows the direct action which occurs when the ion channel is an integral part of the receptor, as in the nicotinic acetylcholine receptor. In (b) and (c) the receptor molecule acts indirectly via activation of a G protein. In (b) the G protein acts directly on the channel to open or close it. In (c) the G protein activates an enzyme which generates a second messenger such as cyclic AMP which itself then alters the state of the channel. (From Aidley, 1998.)

segments. They form part of a large superfamily of receptors, all with seven transmembrane segments. Different members of the super-family respond individually to various neurotransmitters, neuropep-tides, hormones, olfactory stimulants or (for rhodopsin and other visual pigments) the isomerizations of retinal produced by light.

G proteins consist of three subunits, named α, β and γ. At rest they are in the trimeric form $\alpha\beta\gamma$ with guanosine diphosphate (GDP) bound tightly to the α subunit. When a neurotransmitter molecule binds to the receptor, the receptor interacts with the G protein so that it releases the GDP and binds guanosine triphosphate (GTP) in its $\beta\gamma$ subunit. The α subunit then binds to an effector molecule and activates it. Sometimes the $\beta\gamma$ subunit also acts as an activator. Fatty-acid chains attached to the two subunits keep them in contact with

Table 8.1	*Some neurotransmitter receptors*	
Transmitter	Ionotropic	Metabotropic
Acetylcholine	Nicotinic receptors	Muscarinic receptors M_1 to M_5
GABA	$GABA_A$ receptor	$GABA_B$ receptor
Glycine	Glycine receptor	–
5-hydroxytryptamine	5-HT_3 receptor	$5\text{-HT}_{1,2,4}$ receptors
Glutamate receptors	AMPA-kainate receptors NMDA receptors	$mGluR_1$ to $mGluR_5$ receptors
ATP	P_{2X} receptor	P_{2Y} receptor
Noradrenaline	–	$\alpha_1, \alpha_2, \beta_1$ and β_2 receptors
Dopamine	–	D_1-like and D_2-like receptors
Neuropeptides	–	Rhodopsin-like (e.g. substance P, enkephalin) Glucagon-receptor-like (e.g. VIP)

Notes: Abbreviations: GABA, γ-amino butyric acid; 5-HT, 5-hydroxytryptamine; AMPA, α-amino-3-hydroxy-5-methyl-4-isoxazolepropionate; NMDA, N–methyl-D-aspartate; VIP, vasoactive intestinal polypeptide. Ionotropic receptors have their own intrinsic ion channel and mediate fast synaptic transmission. Metabotropic receptors activate ion channels indirectly via G proteins and (usually) second-messenger systems.

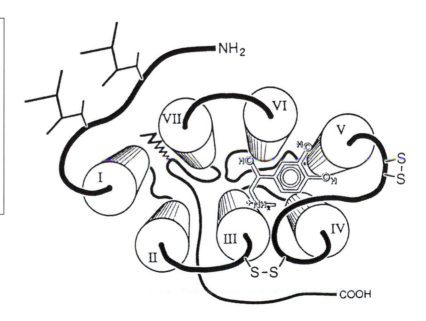

Figure 8.10 The probable arrangement of the transmembrane helices in the β_2-adrenergic receptor, with adrenaline in the binding site. The molecule is drawn as seen from the outer side of the plasma membrane. (From Ostrowski et al., 1992. Reprinted, with permission, from the *Annual Review of Pharmacology and Toxicology*, Volume 32 © 1992 by Annual Reviews www.AnnualReviews.org.)

the plasma membrane, so that they can shuttle between the receptor and the effector molecules.

The effector molecule is sometimes an ion channel, as occurs in the muscarinic action of acetylcholine on the heart. More commonly it is an enzyme whose activation leads to the production of a second messenger. Thus the membrane-bound enzyme adenylyl cyclase is activated by certain G proteins in order to make cyclic AMP from ATP. The cyclic AMP then activates the enzyme protein kinase A, which will result in the phosphorylation of some target molecule such as an ion channel.

An alternative route for G protein action is the phosphatidyl inositol signalling system. Here the G protein activates the enzyme phospholipase C, which hydrolyses the membrane phospholipid phosphatidyl inositol to produce diacyl glycerol and inositol trisphosphate (IP_3). The IP_3 acts as a second messenger by activating Ca^{2+}-release channels in the endoplasmic reticulum membrane, so raising the intracellular Ca^{2+} concentration.

These systems clearly involve some considerable amplification. One receptor molecule binding a single neurotransmitter molecule can activate a number of G-protein molecules, and each activated effector molecule will produce several second-messenger molecules.

8.7 | Electrotonic synapses

An electrotonic synapse is one where the pre-synaptic cell excites the post-synaptic cell directly by means of electric current flow.

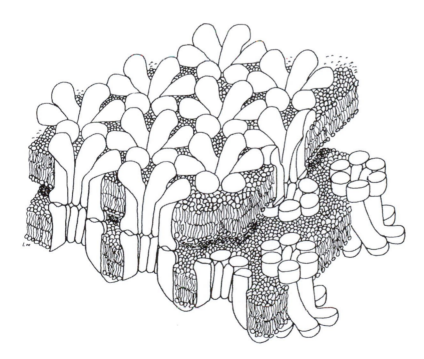

Figure 8.11 The structure of gap junctions, as deduced from X-ray diffraction studies on material isolated from mouse liver cells. (From Makowski *et al.*, 1984.)

Synapses of this type were first discovered in the multi-cellular giant fibres involved in the escape responses of crayfish and earthworms, where they serve to carry the action potential from one cell to another. They also occur between some cells in the central nervous systems of mammals and other animals, where they probably serve to promote synchrony of action in adjacent cells.

Electron microscopy of electrotonic synapses shows regions where the intercellular space between the two cells is much narrower than usual, being about 2 nm instead of 20 nm. These regions are known as 'gap junctions'. They contain channels which provide direct connections between the pre- and post-synaptic cells, so that current can flow readily from one cell to the other. Each gap junction channel is composed of a pair of hexamers, one in each of the two apposed membranes, as is shown in Figure 8.11. The hexamers are known as connexons, and their individual subunits are proteins called connexins.

The mechanism of contraction in skeletal muscle

Skeletal muscles are the engines of the body. They account for over a quarter of its weight and the major part of its energy expenditure. They are attached to the bones of the skeleton and so serve to produce movements or exert forces. Hence they are central to such activities as voluntary movement, maintenance of posture, breathing, eating, directing the gaze and producing gestures and facial expressions. Skeletal muscles are activated by motoneurons, as we have seen in previous chapters. Their cells are elongate and multi-nuclear and the contractile material within them shows cross-striations. Hence skeletal muscle is a form of *striated muscle*. In contrast, cardiac and smooth muscles have cells with single nuclei, and smooth muscles are not striated; we shall examine their properties in Chapters 12 and 13.

9.1 | Anatomy

Skeletal muscle fibres are multi-nucleate cells formed by fusion of elongated uni-nucleate cells called myoblasts whose respective nuclei become arranged around the edge of the fibre. Mature fibres may be as long as the muscle (Figure 9.1) of which they form part, and 10 to 100 μm in diameter. Bundles of muscle fibres are surrounded by a further sheet of connective tissue, the perimysium, and the whole muscle is contained within an outer sheet of tough connective tissue, the epimysium. These connective tissue sheets are continuous with the insertions and tendons which serve to attach the muscles to the skeleton. An excellent blood supply provides a network of blood capillaries between individual fibres.

The structural components of each muscle fibre reflect both its excitable and its contractile functions. The muscle fibre is bounded by its cell membrane, sometimes called the sarcolemma, to which a thin layer of connective tissue, the endomysium, is attached. There are also extensive, specialized, internal membrane systems involved in regulating activation of mechanical activity. Thus, there is a fine system of interconnecting *transverse tubules*

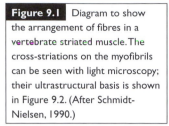

Figure 9.1 Diagram to show the arrangement of fibres in a vertebrate striated muscle. The cross-striations on the myofibrils can be seen with light microscopy; their ultrastructural basis is shown in Figure 9.2. (After Schmidt-Nielsen, 1990.)

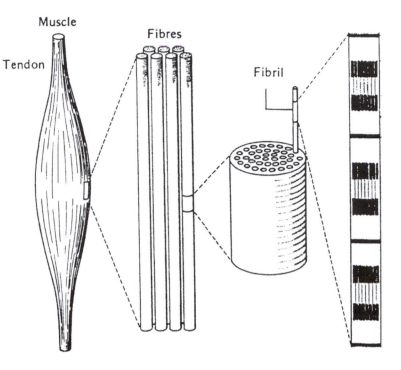

invaginated from the sarcolemma at regularly spaced intervals along the fibre length oriented transversely across the fibre axis. In addition, a *sarcoplasmic reticulum* forms a separate intracellular membrane network of tubes and sacs acting as an intracellular calcium storage site. Muscle cells also contain organelles important in energy metabolism, cell repair and protein synthesis in common with other cells. Mitochondria, lipid and glycogen granules are particularly required in the energy metabolism that sustains contractile activity. Muscle cells also contain ribosomes and lysosomes, and are abundant in a number of specific proteins such as *myoglobin*, which acts as an oxygen store, *creatinine phosphokinase*, which acts to mobilize energy supplies, and *dystrophin*, important in preserving cell membrane integrity, abnormalities in which are implicated in muscular dystrophy.

9.2 | The structure of the myofibril

Most of the remaining fibre interior consists of the protein filaments that constitute the contractile apparatus, grouped together in bundles called *myofibrils*. They have characteristic banding patterns. The bands on adjacent myofibrils are transversely aligned so that the whole fibre appears striated. In order to see the striations by light microscopy it is necessary to fix and stain the fibres, or to use phase-contrast, polarized light or interference microscopy.

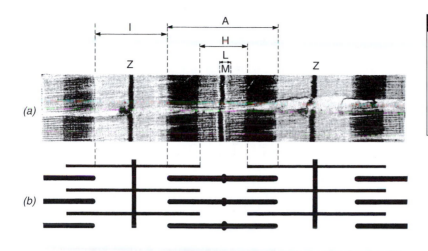

(a)

(b)

Figure 9.2 The striation pattern of a vertebrate skeletal muscle fibre as seen by electron microscopy of thin sections (*a*), and its interpretation as two sets of interdigitating filaments (*b*). (Photograph for (*a*) supplied by Dr H. E. Huxley.)

Figure 9.2*a* shows the striation pattern as seen by these methods and by low-power electron microscopy. The two main bands are the dark, strongly birefringent A band and the lighter, less birefringent I band. These bands alternate along the length of the myofibril. In the middle of each I band is a dark line, the Z line. In the middle of the A band is a lighter region, the H zone, which is bisected by a darker line, the M line. A lighter region in the middle of the H zone, the L zone, can sometimes be distinguished. (These letters used to describe the striation pattern are mostly the initials of names which are now no longer used.) The unit of length between two Z lines is called the *sarcomere*.

In the 1950s the use of the techniques of electron microscopy and thin sectioning, especially by H. E. Huxley and his colleagues, enabled the structural basis of the striation pattern to be discerned (Figures 9.2*b*, 9.3). The myofibrils are composed of two sets of filaments, thick ones about 11 nm in diameter and thin ones about 5 nm in diameter. The thick filaments run the length of the A band. The thin filaments are attached to the Z lines and extend through the I bands into the A bands. The H zone is the region of the A band between the ends of the two sets of thin filaments, and the M line is caused by cross-links between the thick filaments in the middle of the sarcomere. The thick filaments have projections from them except in a short central region which corresponds to the L zone. In the overlap region these projections may be attached to the thin filaments so as to form *cross-bridges* between the two sets of filaments.

The two major proteins of the myofibril are *myosin* and *actin*. When myofibrils are washed in a solution that dissolves myosin the A bands disappear, and further washing with a solution that dissolves actin causes the I bands to disappear. This suggests that the thick filaments are composed largely of myosin and the thin filaments largely of actin. Thin filaments also contain the proteins *tropomyosin* and *troponin*, which are concerned with the control of contraction, as we shall see later.

Figure 9.3 Thin longitudinal section of a glycerol-extracted rabbit psoas muscle fibre. Notice, particularly, the cross-bridges between the thick and thin filaments. (Photograph supplied by Dr H. E. Huxley.)

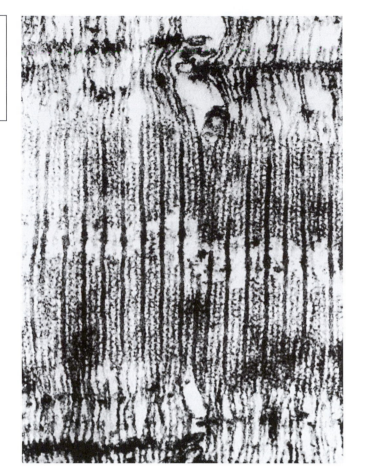

Figure 9.4 The locations of titin and nebulin within the sarcomere. Nebulin is associated with the thin filaments. Each titin molecule is attached at one end to the Z line and at its other end is bound to a thick filament; the section in the I band is highly extensible. (From Bagshaw, 1993, *Muscle Contraction*, Figure 4.16, p. 56, with kind permission from Kluwer Academic Publishers.)

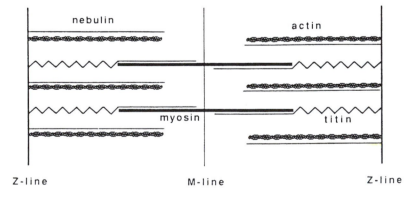

The Z line contains the protein α-*actinin*, which binds to the actin filaments. Two large filamentous proteins also occur in the myofibril: *nebulin*, which runs parallel to the thin filaments, and *titin*, which runs from the Z line to near the middle of the sarcomere and is bound to the thick filaments in the A band (Figure 9.4). Titin is a very large molecule (molecular weight about 3 million) and very elastic; it probably serves to keep the thick filaments in the middle of the sarcomere when the myofibril is stretched.

9.3 | The sliding-filament theory

Prior to 1954, most suggestions as to the mechanism of muscular contraction involved the coiling and contraction of long protein molecules, rather like the shortening of a helical spring. In that year the *sliding-filament theory* was independently formulated by H. E. Huxley and Jean Hanson, using phase-contrast microscopy of myofibrils from glycerol-extracted muscles, and by A. F. Huxley and R. Niedergerke, using interference microscopy of living muscle fibres. In each case the authors showed that the A band does not change in length either when the muscle is stretched or when it shortens actively or passively. This suggests that contraction is brought about by movement of the thin filaments between the thick filaments. The sliding is thought to be caused by a series of cyclic reactions between the projections on the myosin filaments and active sites on the actin filaments; each projection first attaches itself to the actin filament to form a cross-bridge, then pulls on it and finally releases it, moving back to attach to another site further along the actin filament.

Let us now have a look at some of the further evidence for this theory.

9.3.1 The lengths of the filaments

Electron microscopy provides evidence that the filaments do not change in length when the muscle is stretched or allowed to shorten. This is just what we would expect if such length changes involve sliding of the filaments past each other. Measurements on frog muscles suggest that the thick filaments are 1.6 μm long, and that the thin filaments extend for 1.0 μm on each side of the Z line.

Electron microscopy has to be performed on muscle tissue which has been fixed and stained. There is a need, therefore, for some length-measuring method which can be applied directly to the living muscle. This is provided by the technique of X-ray diffraction, in which a beam of X-rays is passed through a muscle and the resulting diffraction pattern indicates the distances between repeat units in the muscle structure.

In the thick filaments the X-ray diffraction pattern suggests that there are structures which repeat axially at 14.3 nm and helically at 42.9 nm. In the thin filaments there seem to be structures arranged on helices with pitches of 5.1, 5.9 and about 37 nm.

The structural basis of these repeat distances we shall return to later. What is important in our present context is that they do not change when the muscle is lengthened or shortened, either when it is resting or during contraction. This provides further evidence that the filaments themselves do not shorten or lengthen during the corresponding changes in muscle length.

9.3.2 The relation between sarcomere length and isometric tension

The suggestion that contraction depends on the interaction of the actin and myosin filaments at the cross-bridges implies that the isometric tension should be proportional to the degree of overlap of the filaments. In order to test this idea it is necessary to measure the active increment of isometric tension at different known sarcomere lengths. The measurements have to be done on a single fibre and there are some technical difficulties because sarcomeres at the ends of a fibre may take up lengths different from those in the middle. A. F. Huxley and his colleagues overcame these difficulties by building an apparatus which used optical servomechanisms to maintain the sarcomere lengths in the middle of a fibre constant during a contraction.

Figure 9.5 summarizes the results of these experiments. It is evident that the length–tension diagram consists of a series of straight lines connected by a short curved region. There is a 'plateau' of constant tension at sarcomere lengths between 2.05 and 2.2 μm. Above this range tension falls linearly with increasing length; the projected line through most of the points in this region reaches zero at 3.65 μm. Below the plateau, tension falls gradually with decreasing length down to about 1.65 μm, then much more steeply, reaching zero at about 1.3 μm.

Does this curve fit the predictions of the sliding-filament theory? We need to know the dimensions of the filaments (Figure 9.6). Measurements by electron microscopy indicate that the myosin filaments are 1.6 μm long and the actin filaments, including the Z line, are 2.05 μm long. The middle region of the myosin filaments, which is bare of projections and therefore cannot form cross-bridges, is 0.15 to 0.2 μm long and the thickness of the Z line is about 0.05 μm.

Now let us see if the length–tension diagram shown in Figure 9.5 can be related to these dimensions, starting at long sarcomere

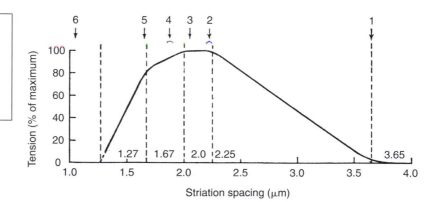

Figure 9.5 The isometric tension (active increment) of a frog muscle fibre at different sarcomere lengths. The numbers 1 to 6 refer to the myofilament positions shown in Figure 9.7. (From Gordon *et al.*, 1966.)

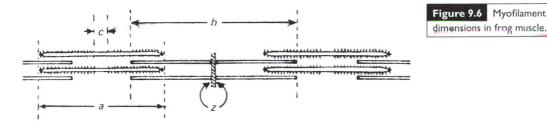

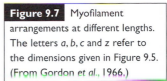

Figure 9.6 Myofilament dimensions in frog muscle.

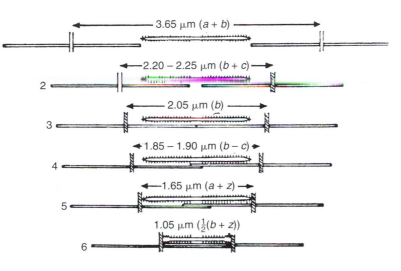

Figure 9.7 Myofilament arrangements at different lengths. The letters a, b, c and z refer to the dimensions given in Figure 9.5. (From Gordon et al., 1966.)

lengths and working through to short ones. Above 3.65 μm (stage 1 in Figure 9.7) there should be no cross-bridges formed, and therefore no tension development. In fact there is some tension development up to about 3.8 μm; this might well be due to some residual irregularities in the system. Between 3.65 μm and 2.2 to 2.25 μm (stages 1 to 2) the number of cross-bridges increases linearly with decrease in length, and therefore the isometric tension should show a similar increase. It does. With further shortening (stages 2 to 3) the number of cross-bridges remains constant and therefore there should be a plateau of constant tension in this region. There is. After stage 3 we might expect there to be some increase in the internal resistance to shortening since the actin filaments must now overlap, and after stage 4 the actin filaments from one half of the sarcomere might interfere with the cross-bridge formation in the other half of the sarcomere. We would expect both these effects to reduce the isometric tension, which does indeed fall at lengths below 2.0 μm. At 1.65 μm (stage 5) the myosin filaments will hit the Z line, and so there should be a considerable increase in the resistance to further shortening; there is a distinct kink in the curve at almost exactly this point, after which the tension falls much more sharply. The curve reaches zero tension at about 1.3 μm, before stage 6 is reached.

It would be difficult to find a more precise test of the sliding-filament theory than is given by this experiment, and the theory clearly passes the test with flying colours.

9.4 | The molecular basis of contraction

We have seen that the myofibrils contain a small number of different proteins. Of these myosin and actin are the most important since they are involved in the splitting of ATP and the process of contraction.

9.4.1 Myosin

Myosin (Figure 9.8) is a rather complex molecule with a molecular weight of about 470 000 Da. It is made up of six polypeptide chains, two long ones (heavy chains) and four short ones (light chains). Electron microscopy of isolated molecules shows that they consist of two 'heads' attached to a long 'tail'. The two heavy chains wind round each other to form the tail region, but they separate to form the two heads. The light chains, of two types called the essential and regulatory light chains, form part of the heads.

A most important property of myosin is that it is an ATPase, i.e. it acts as an enzyme to hydrolyse ATP, forming ADP and inorganic phosphate. Treatment with the proteolytic enzyme trypsin splits the myosin molecule into two sections known as light meromyosin and heavy meromyosin; only heavy meromyosin acts as an ATPase. Electron microscopy shows that heavy meromyosin has two 'heads' and a short 'tail', whereas light meromyosin is a rod-like molecule. Heavy meromyosin can be further split by digestion by papain, to give two globular S1 subfragments (the 'heads') and a short rod-like S2 subfragment. The ATPase activity is confined to the S1 subfragment. Light meromyosin molecules will aggregate to form filaments under suitable conditions, but neither heavy meromyosin nor its two subfragments will.

H. E. Huxley found that under the right conditions myosin molecules can aggregate to form filaments. These filaments have regularly spaced projections on them which almost certainly

Figure 9.8 The six polypeptide chains that form the myosin molecule. The whole molecule consists of two globular heads attached to a long tail. The tail or rod is a coiled-coil formed from the α-helical regions of the two heavy chains; it is divided into an LMM (light meromyosin) section, and an S2 (subfragment 2) section. Each heavy chain has a globular region that combines with two light chains to form an S1 head. The light chains are of two types, called essential (ELC) and regulatory (RLC). Heavy meromyosin (HMM) consists of the S1 and S2 subfragments. Enzymic activity and the molecular motor are found in the S1 heads. LMM aggregates with others to form the backbone of the myosin filament, and the S2 part of the rod connects it to the two S1 heads. (Reprinted from *Trends in Biochemical Sciences*, **19**, I. Rayment and H. M. Holden, The three-dimensional structure of a molecular motor, p. 129, copyright 1994, with permission from Elsevier Science.)

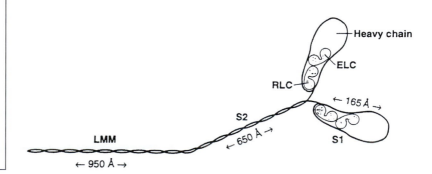

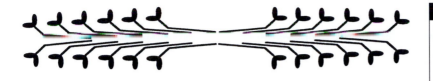

Figure 9.9 How the myosin molecules assemble to form a thick filament with a projection-free shaft in the middle and reversed polarity of the molecules in each half of the sarcomere. (From Bagshaw, 1993, *Muscle Contraction*, Figure 4.7, p. 43, with kind permission from Kluwer Academic Publications.)

correspond to the projections and cross-bridges seen in thin sections of myofibrils. In the middle of each filament is a section from which these projections were absent, which must correspond to the L zone of intact muscle fibres. Similar filaments could be isolated from homogenised myofibrils; they were all 1.6 μm long, whereas the 'artificial' filaments were variable in length. Huxley suggested that the 'tails' of the myosin molecules become attached to each other to form a filament, as shown in Figure 9.9, with the 'heads' projecting from the body of the filament. Notice particularly that this arrangement accounts for the bare region in the middle, and also that it implies that the polarity of the myosin molecules is reversed in the two halves of the filament.

X-ray diffraction studies show that there is an axial repeat of 14.3 nm and a helical repeat of 42.9 nm on the myosin filament, as has already been mentioned. This suggests that a group of myosin heads emerges from the filament every 14.3 nm, and that their orientation rotates so that every third group is in line. There are probably three myosin molecules in each group, as is suggested in Figure 9.10*a*.

The amino-acid sequence of the myosin heavy chain suggests that the whole of the tail section of the molecule is α-helical in structure, with the two heavy chains coiled round each other. The S1 head has a much less regular structure. X-ray diffraction studies by Rayment and his colleagues show that the head is divided into various functional regions: an actin-binding site, an ATP-binding site and a lever arm about 10 nm long, which connects to the S2 link (see Figure 9.11). The light chains are associated with the lever arm section of the S1 head.

9.4.2 Actin

Isolated actin exists in two forms: G-actin, a more or less globular molecule of molecular weight about 42 000, and F-actin, a fibrous protein which is a polymer of G-actin. Neither form has any ATPase activity, but they will both combine with myosin. F-actin consists of two chains of monomers connected together in the form of a double helix, as is shown in Figure 9.10*b*. The thin filaments in intact muscle also contain tropomyosin and troponin, probably arranged as in Figure 9.10*c*.

9.4.3 The interaction of actin, myosin and ATP

If solutions of actin and myosin are mixed, a great increase in viscosity occurs, due to the formation of a complex called *actomyosin*. Actomyosin is an ATPase which is activated by Mg^{2+} ions. 'Pure'

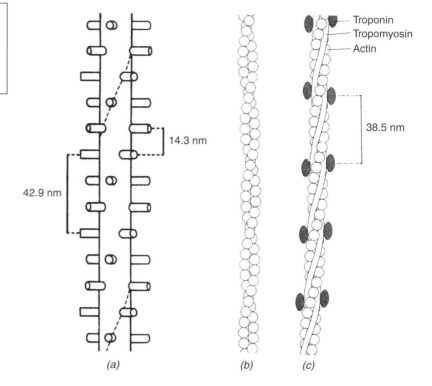

Figure 9.10 Models of the structure of the thick and thin filaments: (*a*) the myosin filament; (*b*) F-actin; (*c*) the thin filament. (Based on Offer (1974) after various authors.)

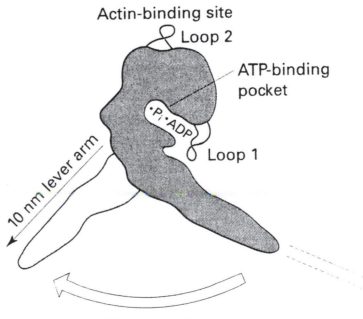

Figure 9.11 The swinging lever arm model for S1 action. A change in shape of the molecule near to the ATP-binding pocket produces a movement of about 10 nm at the end of the lever arm. This pulls on the S2 link, which is attached to the myosin filament backbone. (Redrawn after Spudich (1994), with permission from the author and *Nature*, Macmillan Magazines Limited.)

actomyosin (a mixture of purified actin and purified myosin) will split ATP in the absence of Ca^{2+} ions. However 'natural' actomyosin (an actomyosin-like complex which can be extracted from minced muscle with strong salt solutions, and which also contains tropomyosin and troponin) can only split ATP if there is a low concentration of Ca^{2+} ions present. In the absence of Ca^{2+} ions, addition of ATP to a solution of natural actomyosin results in a decrease in viscosity, suggesting that the actin–myosin complex becomes dissociated.

We can use these observations to make plausible suggestions about how actin and myosin interact within the filament array in which they exist in the living muscle. In the resting condition there is an adequate concentration of ATP and a very low concentration of Ca^{2+}, so there is no interaction between the actin and myosin and no ATP splitting. On activation the Ca^{2+} concentration rises and so cross-bridges are formed between the two sets of filaments, ATP is split and sliding occurs.

In recent years we have learnt much more about the myosin motor and its interaction with actin from some remarkable experiments involving *in vitro* motility assays. These use purified actin and myosin in systems that allow the movement of single filaments to be seen by light microscopy. One arrangement is shown in Figure 9.12: an actin filament to which a fluorescent dye has been attached is placed on a 'lawn' of myosin S1 heads. In the absence of ATP the actin filament is bound to the S1 heads, but there is no movement. On adding ATP the actin moves across the lawn at a speed comparable with the sliding of filaments in whole muscle.

The primary source of the movement is probably a change in shape of the myosin S1 head, brought about by the splitting of ATP, so that the lever arm section swings through about 10 nm and thereby pulls on the S2 link and so on the whole myosin filament (Figure 9.11). Fine evidence for this 'swinging lever' model comes from some experiments by Spudich and his colleagues (1995) in which S1 mutants with lever arms longer or shorter than usual were used in a motility assay: the velocities of the actin filaments were proportional to the lengths of the lever arm.

Cross-bridge action is thus a cyclical process. Each cross-bridge will attach to the adjacent actin filament, its lever arm will swing so as to pull the actin and myosin filaments past each other, then it will detach from the actin filament. The cross-bridge is then ready to attach to a new site on the actin filament and so repeat the cycle.

Figure 9.12 Diagram to show an actin filament moving on a lawn of myosin S1 heads in an *in vitro* motility assay. The direction of sliding is determined by the polarity of the actin filament. ATP is split in the process. (From H. E. Huxley (1990), reproduced with permission of the American Society for Biochemistry and Molecular Biology.)

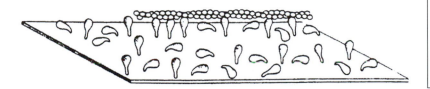

The energy for each turn of the cycle is provided by the breakdown of one molecule of ATP to ADP and inorganic phosphate.

9.4.4   The molecular basis of activation

As mentioned earlier, pure actin will react with pure myosin so as to split ATP in the absence of Ca^{2+} ions. But if tropomyosin and troponin are also present, the actin–myosin interaction and ATP splitting will occur in the presence of Ca^{2+} ions. Hence it is probable that tropomyosin and troponin are intimately involved in the control of muscular contraction.

Tropomyosin is a fibrous protein which will bind to actin and troponin. Troponin is a globular protein with three subunits: one binds to actin, another to tropomyosin and a third combines reversibly with Ca^{2+} ions, undergoing a conformational change in the process.

The molecular ratios of actin, tropomyosin and troponin in the muscle are 7:1:1. A model of the thin filament incorporating these ratios is shown in Figure 9.10c, where the tropomyosin molecules lie in the grooves between the two chains of actin monomers and a troponin molecule is attached with each tropomyosin molecule to every seventh actin monomer. This arrangement would give a repeat distance of $(7 \times 5.5) = 38.5$ nm for the troponin and tropomyosin, which agrees well with the observation of X-ray reflections at this distance.

Evidence about the structure of the thin filament under different conditions has been obtained from X-ray diffraction measurements

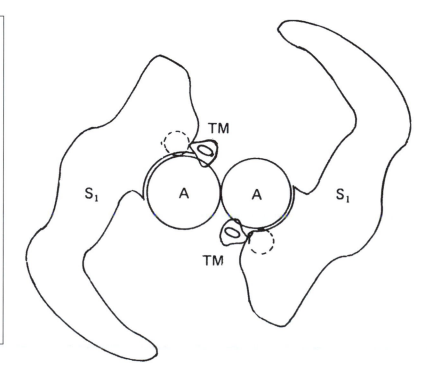

Figure 9.13 One of the models proposed to show how movement of tropomyosin molecules may affect actin–myosin interactions. A thin filament is seen in cross-section with actin (A) and tropomyosin (TM) molecules. Two myosin S_1 subunits are shown attached to the thin filaments. Tropomyosin positions are shown for the muscle at rest (dotted circle) and when active (contours). Other models give somewhat different shapes and positions for the various protein molecules, but all agree that the tropomyosin molecule moves into the 'groove' between the actin monomers on activation. It is thought that the S_1 heads are unable to attach to the actin filament until this movement takes place. (From Huxley, 1976.)

and from computer analysis simulating optical diffraction of electron micrographs. It seems likely that the binding of Ca^{2+} by a troponin molecule causes a change in its shape which draws the tropomyosin molecule to which it is attached further into the groove between the two chains of actin monomers (Figure 9.13). In the resting condition it looks as though the tropomyosin molecules prevent actin–myosin interaction by covering the myosin binding sites on the actin monomers. So this movement on activation has the exciting consequence that each tropomyosin molecule uncovers the myosin-binding sites on seven actin monomers. The myosin heads can then combine with the actin and so the muscle contracts. It is a very elegant piece of biological machinery.

10

The activation of skeletal muscle

Skeletal muscle contraction is ultimately initiated by activity in the nervous system. Muscle receives both sensory and motor nerve fibres. The sensory nerves convey information about the state of the muscle to the nervous system. This includes information about muscle length detected by the muscle spindles and tension detected by the Golgi tendon organs. There are also a variety of free nerve endings in the muscle tissue, some of which convey sensations of pain. Of the motor fibres in mammals, the γ-motoneurons provide a separate motor nerve supply for the muscle fibres of the muscle spindles. However, the bulk of the muscle fibres are supplied by the α-motoneurons. Each α-motoneuron innervates a number of muscle fibres, from less than ten in the extraocular muscles, which move the eyeball in its socket, to over a thousand in a large limb muscle. The complex of one motoneuron plus the muscle fibres which it innervates is called a *motor unit*. Since they are all activated by the same nerve cell, all the muscle fibres in a single motor unit contract at the same time. However, muscle fibres belonging to different motor units may well contract at different times. Thus, most mammalian muscle fibres are contacted by a single nerve terminal, although sometimes there may be two terminals originating from the same nerve axon. Muscle fibres of this type are known as *twitch fibres*, since they respond to nervous stimulation with a rapid twitch. In the frog and other lower vertebrates another type of muscle fibre is commonly found, in which there are a large number of nerve terminals on each muscle fibre. These are known as *tonic fibres*, since their contractions are slow and maintained. There are some tonic fibres in the extraocular muscles of mammals, and also in the muscles of the larynx and the middle ear.

10.1 Ion channels in the membrane of skeletal muscle

The excitable properties of muscle membranes resemble those of nerve cell membranes in a number of important respects. Their surface membranes also contain sodium channels. However, muscle membranes contain at least three, rather than a single, potassium channel type. One is activated by depolarization over a time course close to that found in nerve membranes, and a second is activated over considerably longer time courses of hundreds of milliseconds. Finally, an inward rectification channel allows K^+ to pass more easily into than out of the cell, thereby minimizing leak currents and reducing the inward current required to maintain or depolarize the resting potential.

Skeletal muscle also shows a significant Cl^- conductance not found in nerve. There is no evidence that Cl^- is actively transported across cell membranes. Consequently, this ion is distributed passively across the membrane according to the Nernst equation applied to Cl^-, assuming a potential equal to the resting potential. In turn this resulting distribution of Cl^- tends to stabilize the membrane potential at its resting level (Ferenczi et al., 2004). Deficiencies or absences of functioning chloride channels result in the unwanted repetitive action-potential firing characteristic of the clinical condition *myotonia congenita* (Adrian and Bryant, 1974).

Finally, skeletal muscle also contains calcium channels in their transverse tubular membranes. In invertebrate muscles, these give rise to the inward currents that are responsible for the action potential, as well as initiating the contraction process itself. However the currents they produce activate too slowly to either contribute to normal electrical properties or initiate contraction in vertebrate skeletal muscle. However, as will be explained below, the channels may instead simply act as voltage sensors that initiate further processes leading to contractile activation. Nevertheless they are important in action-potential generation in mammalian cardiac muscle (Chapter 12). Furthermore, abnormal Ca^{2+} permeability properties may contribute to the pathological changes observed in dystrophic muscle.

10.2 | Action potential generation in surface and tubular membranes of skeletal muscle

Activation of the motoneuron that innervates the muscle fibres making up its motor unit initiates an action potential that is propagated down its axon to neuromuscular junctions with the individual muscle fibres in the same motor unit. The resulting release of transmitter causes post-synaptic depolarization (see Chapter 7). This in turn results in an action potential that propagates over the surface membrane of the skeletal muscle fibre. As indicated in Chapter 9, skeletal muscle contains an additional, transverse tubular system formed from invaginations of the cell surface membrane whose lumina communicate with the extracellular space.

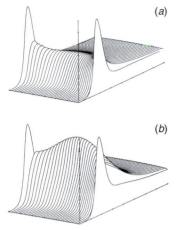

(a)

(b)

Figure 10.1 Action potential
generation in the surface and
transverse tubular membranes
of amphibian skeletal muscle. The
vertical axis represents membrane
potential change resulting from
action potentials plotted against
the horizontal time axis running to
the right. These are represented
through the surface membrane
and transverse tubules, along
the cross-section of the fibre, of
diameter 50 microns represented
along the horizontal distance
axis running to the left. In (a) the
regenerative activity propagating
along the length of the surface
membrane is permitted to spread
passively into a transverse tubular
system modelled without sodium
channels. In (b) the presence
of tubular sodium channels
results in an inward propagation
of regenerative activity, and a
successful tubular excitation.
In both (a) and (b) tubular and
surface membranes are separated
by a 150 Ω cm² access resistance.
(From Adrian and Peachey, 1973.)

A rapid propagation of the action potential along the surface
membrane is essential for a prompt spread of excitation from the
neuromuscular junction to the ends of the fibre. However, as will
become apparent below, depolarization of the tubular system whose
membranes are normally continuous with those of the surface is
essential for initiation of the contractile activity itself. Detachment
of the transverse tubules by an osmotic shock produced by an introduction and withdrawal of extracellular glycerol (Fraser *et al.*, 1998)
thus abolishes contractile activation despite leaving surface electrical activity intact.

Such a requirement for tubular excitation carries its own implications for membrane function. Firstly, R. H. Adrian and Peachey
(1973) demonstrated that a passive excitation of tubular membranes
by a surface action potential would be unlikely to successfully initiate contraction, particularly in membranes in the depths of the tubular system. Figure 10.1*a* illustrates this, showing the surface action
potentials at the edges of the block diagram, and the resulting passive spread of tubular excitation in traces between these. Secondly,
the presence of the transverse tubular membranes results in five to
tenfold higher membrane capacitance referred to unit muscle compared to axonal surface membranes. This would markedly slow the
velocity of conduction (see Chapter 6) of the action potential propagating along the surface of the muscle fibre.

These problems are overcome in the membrane system of skeletal
muscle first through a presence of activatable sodium channels within
the transverse tubular system. These would occur at a density sufficient to generate action potential activity following excitation from
the surface, but not to themselves influence the voltage across the
membrane surface. Sodium channels thus also occur in the tubular
membranes, but at a lower density than on the surface. Second, there
is evidence for an existence of partial luminal constrictions restricting
electrical access to the tubular lumina. Such a situation is illustrated in
Figure 10.1*b*. It results in action-potential generation and consequent
excitation of the entire tubular system following surface excitation.

Such an access resistance would direct local-circuit currents along
the membrane surface rather than the partially isolated tubular system. This would maximize the velocity of propagation of the surface
action potential, whilst permitting sufficient local-circuit current to
initiate tubular action potentials as the propagating surface action
potential passes each successive tubular opening. Findings by Sheikh
et al. (2001) indeed fulfilled predictions for such a partial tubular
isolation. Thus detachment of the transverse tubules by osmotic
shock paradoxically leaves the surface conduction velocity intact.
Furthermore, immunological localization of sodium-channel densities localized these selectively to the peripheries of the transverse
tubular systems, where such excitation would be most effective.

The partial tubular isolation would also permit tubular action
potentials with time courses that could potentially substantially differ from those on the surface. This may be reflected in the prolonged

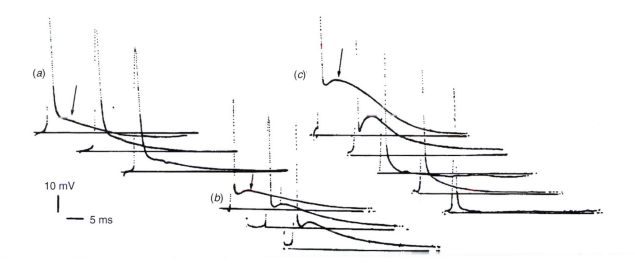

after-depolarizations (arrowed) following the initial action potential upstroke and recovery illustrated in Figure 10.2a, b. These become more prominent with increases in temperature, likely reflecting the temperature sensitivity of an active rather than a passive process. However, further increases in temperature further increasing surface action-potential conduction velocities would shorten their transit times in any given membrane region. This should eventually result in a failure of tubular excitation and an all-or-none disappearance of the delayed tubular wave. Such a prediction was indeed achieved, as shown in Figure 10.2c (Padmanabhan and Huang, 1990).

However, such an isolation of the transverse tubular lumina results in the formation of a restricted extracellular space with which diffusion equilibration with the rest of the extracellular fluid is relatively slow. This would result in a site in which ions may accumulate or from which they may be depleted. They are thus regions for accumulation of K^+ released into the tubular lumina during action-potential firing. This could lead to alterations in excitable properties following the repetitive action-potential firing that accompanies sustained muscle activity during exercise, as will be discussed in Chapter 11. However, recent evidence suggests a lower density of potassium channels in the tubular membrane than in the surface membrane that may minimize this.

Figure 10.2 Surface and tubular (arrowed) components of the muscle fibre action potentials (a). A 4 °C temperature increase shortens the initial peak, but results in more prominent after-potentials with noticeable rising phases (b). However, further warming results in an all-or-nothing disappearance of the delayed tubular wave (c). (From Padmanabhan and Huang, 1990.)

10.3 | Excitation–contraction coupling in skeletal muscle

Such action-potential generation is the likely trigger for contractile activation in skeletal muscle. Excitation–contraction coupling refers to the sequence of events that intervene between action-potential activation and initiation of tension generation by the actin and myosin filaments. The immediate trigger for excitation–contraction

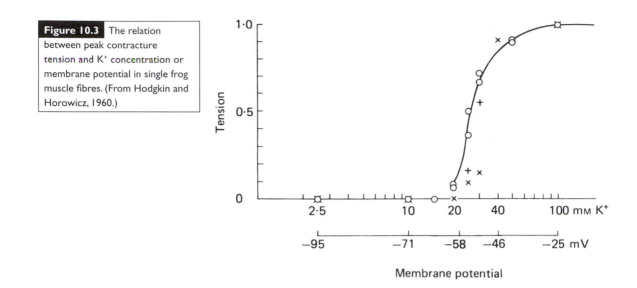

Figure 10.3 The relation between peak contracture tension and K⁺ concentration or membrane potential in single frog muscle fibres. (From Hodgkin and Horowicz, 1960.)

coupling is likely the membrane-potential change resulting from the electrical excitation. It thus can be reproduced by experimental manipulations of the resting potential. Thus, when muscle fibres are immersed in a solution containing a high concentration of K⁺ that depolarizes the membrane potential (Chapter 3) they undergo a relatively prolonged contraction called a *potassium contracture*. In contrast to the all-or-nothing nature of the action potential, the tension produced is graded with the potassium concentration in a sigmoidal way, as shown in Figure 10.3. Thus, depolarization constitutes an adequate stimulus for contraction. This activation process has distinct physiological properties and kinetics. Although a single action potential along a muscle fibre elicits a single twitch, this persists well beyond its termination, around 50 ms in fast muscle and up to several hundred milliseconds in slow muscle. Furthermore, whereas repetitive stimulation produces a train of action potentials, where these occur above a critical frequency, they result in a fusion of such individual twitches into a sustained and augmented tension generation or *tetanus*. These critical frequencies vary between 300 s⁻¹ for fast muscles down to about 40 s⁻¹ for slow muscles. Furthermore, in addition to various drugs which depolarize the cell membrane, such as acetylcholine and veratridine, contractures can also be produced by agents that do not result in depolarization, including caffeine, likely reflecting actions on later stages in the coupling process.

10.4 | Involvement of Ca²⁺ ions in excitation–contraction coupling

Membrane depolarization is thought to result in a release of intracellularly stored calcium from the sarcoplasmic reticulum. This elevates free cytosolic calcium concentrations that in turn activate the contractile proteins and initiate mechanical activity. Thus, myofibrils can be isolated from muscle by homogenizing the cells followed by differential centrifugation of the homogenate. Such a myofibrillar fraction will split ATP, just as occurs in the contracting muscle, but only in the presence of Ca^{2+}. The concentration of Ca^{2+} required is about 10^{-6} M. This level is low, but not negligible; it is higher than the free Ca^{2+} concentration in the sarcoplasm of the resting muscle of ~100 nM.

This observation suggests a way in which muscular contraction might be controlled: depolarization might cause an increase in the intracellular Ca^{2+} concentration which would then activate the contractile apparatus. Direct evidence for this idea was provided by Ashley and Ridgeway (1968). They used the protein aequorin, isolated from a bioluminescent jellyfish, which emits light in the presence of Ca^{2+} ions. Solutions of aequorin were injected into the large muscle fibres of the barnacle, *Balanus nubilis*. When such a fibre was stimulated electrically it produced a faint glow of light, indicating the presence of free Ca^{2+} ions in its interior. The light output could be measured by using a photomultiplier tube, with the results shown in Figure 10.4. Notice that the time course of the 'Ca^{2+} transient' is a little slower than that of the depolarization, but much faster than that of the ensuing tension change.

Further studies quantifying such Ca^{2+} transients introduced absorbence dyes such as arsenazo III or antipyrylazo III to measure cytoplasmic Ca^{2+} concentrations in amphibian muscle subject to voltage clamp steps (Kovacs *et al.*, 1979). These demonstrated a distinct activation threshold at test voltages around –40 mV. Further depolarization produced steep increases in Ca^{2+} release. Even small,

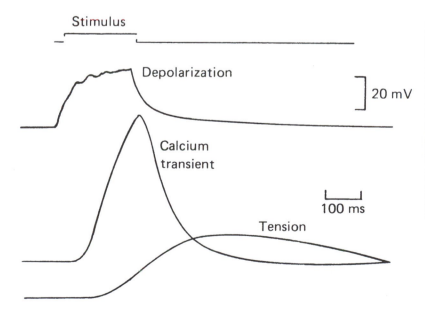

Stimulus

Depolarization

20 mV

Calcium transient

100 ms

Tension

Figure 10.4 Ca^{2+} transient in a barnacle muscle fibre, measured by the aequorin technique. The top trace monitors the stimulus pulse, and the second trace shows the ensuing depolarization. The third trace shows the photomultiplier output, indicating the concentration of free Ca^{2+} ions inside the muscle cell. Finally the bottom trace shows the tension developed. (After Ashley and Ridgeway (1968) redrawn.)

~1.9 mV, changes in test potential resulted in e-fold increases in peak ionized Ca²⁺ concentration (Maylie *et al.*, 1987). However, the Ca²⁺ transients attained a maximum, saturating amplitude at positive voltages. They then persisted even with strong depolarization to test voltages of +170 mV or extracellular Ca²⁺ chelation by EGTA. Both these latter manoeuvres would reduce the inward driving force for Ca²⁺. Furthermore, skeletal muscle remains able to contract in the absence of external Ca²⁺. Together these findings attribute Ca²⁺ transients in skeletal muscle to a release of intracellularly stored calcium through a triggering process independent of extracellular Ca²⁺ entry, but saturating at strongly positive voltages. The elevation in the cytosolic Ca²⁺ concentration in skeletal muscle thus almost entirely reflects its release from such sarcoplasmic reticular stores, with no significant contribution from Ca²⁺ influx from the extracellular space. This release of intracellularly stored Ca²⁺ ions ultimately initiates mechanical activity through their binding to the regulatory protein troponin (Chapter 9).

10.5 | Internal membrane systems

The next question that arises is how does excitation at the cell surface cause release of Ca²⁺ ions inside the fibre? The first step in the solution of this problem was the demonstration by A. F. Huxley and Taylor (1958) that there is a specific inward-conducting mechanism located at the Z line in frog sartorius muscles. The muscle fibres were viewed by polarized light microscopy so as to make the striation pattern visible. They were stimulated by passing depolarizing current through an external microelectrode applied to the fibre surface. The stimulus was effective only when the electrode was positioned at certain 'active spots' located on the fibre surface in rows opposite the Z lines. In these cases the A bands adjacent to the I band opposite the electrode were drawn together, as is shown in Figure 10.5.

At first it was thought that the inward-conducting mechanism was the Z line itself, but on repeating the experiments with crab muscle fibres it was found that the 'active spots' were localized not at the Z line, but near the boundary between the A and I bands. This suggests that there is some transverse structure located at the Z lines in frog muscles and at the A–I boundary in crab muscles.

Figure 10.5 The effect of local depolarizations on a frog muscle fibre. When the electrode is opposite certain active spots in the I band, as shown here, contraction ensues. (Based on Huxley and Taylor, 1958.)

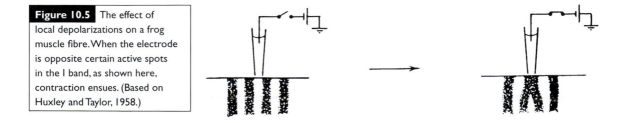

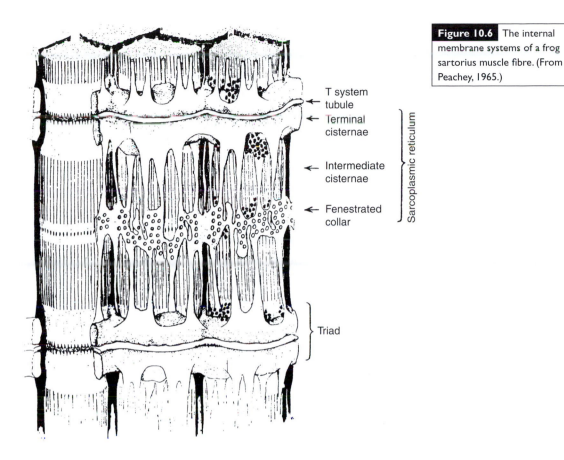

T system tubule

Terminal cisternae

Intermediate cisternae

Fenestrated collar

Sarcoplasmic reticulum

Triad

Figure 10.6 The internal membrane systems of a frog sartorius muscle fibre. (From Peachey, 1965.)

Such a structure was found in the electron microscopic examination of the sarcoplasmic reticulum in various skeletal muscles. This consists of a network of vesicular elements surrounding the myofibrils (Figure 10.6). At the Z lines in frog muscles, and at the A–I boundaries in most other striated muscles, including crab muscles, are structures known as 'triads', in which a central tubular element is situated between two vesicular elements. These central elements of the triads are in fact tubules which run transversely across the fibre and are the transverse (T) tubular system whose electrical properties are discussed in Section 10.2. There is no continuity between the insides of the tubules of the T system and the vesicles of this junctional sarcoplasmic reticulum, although their membranes come into close proximity. The T system tubules open to the exterior at a limited number of sites corresponding to Huxley and Taylor's 'active spots'.

10.6 | Triggering molecules for the release of sarcoplasmic reticular calcium

Triggering of Ca^{2+} release thus entails a transduction of the depolarization in the transverse tubules to a release of Ca^{2+} stored in the sarcoplasmic reticulum. The transverse tubules are most closely associated with the sarcoplasmic reticulum at the 'triads' described by Porter and Palade (1957). Triads consist of two terminal cisternae of the sarcoplasmic reticulum flanking opposite sides of the slightly flattened T tubule. Electron microscopy reveals that these membrane structures appear connected by an array of structures called 'feet', subsequently shown to be anchored in the sarcoplasmic reticulum membrane and consisting of four subunits. The T tubule membrane contains particles grouped in fours ('tetrads') that are positioned opposite the feet. Detailed characterization of these structures (Figure 10.7) by Block *et al.* (1988) revealed two sets of ion channels. The tetrads are groups of four voltage-gated calcium channels, also known as dihydropyridine receptors, since they bind pharmacological agents which are dihydropyridine derivatives.

It has been recently shown that the foot processes are largely made up of the cytoplasmic components of a membrane protein

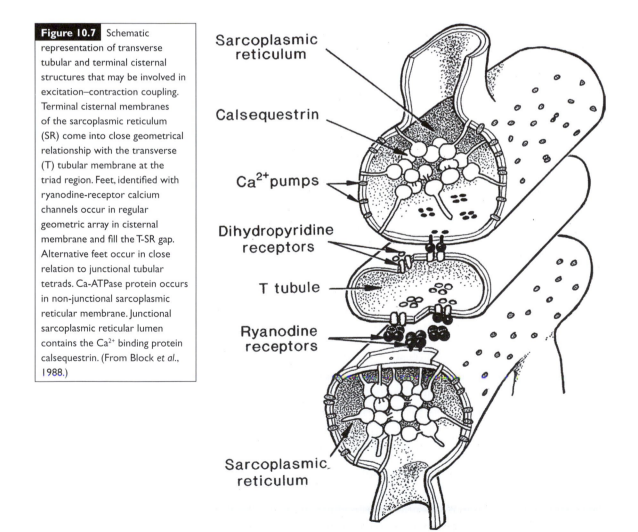

Figure 10.7 Schematic representation of transverse tubular and terminal cisternal structures that may be involved in excitation–contraction coupling. Terminal cisternal membranes of the sarcoplasmic reticulum (SR) come into close geometrical relationship with the transverse (T) tubular membrane at the triad region. Feet, identified with ryanodine-receptor calcium channels occur in regular geometric array in cisternal membrane and fill the T-SR gap. Alternative feet occur in close relation to junctional tubular tetrads. Ca-ATPase protein occurs in non-junctional sarcoplasmic reticular membrane. Junctional sarcoplasmic reticular lumen contains the Ca^{2+} binding protein calsequestrin. (From Block *et al.*, 1988.)

Sarcoplasmic reticulum

Calsequestrin

Ca^{2+} pumps

Dihydropyridine receptors

T tubule

Ryanodine receptors

Sarcoplasmic reticulum

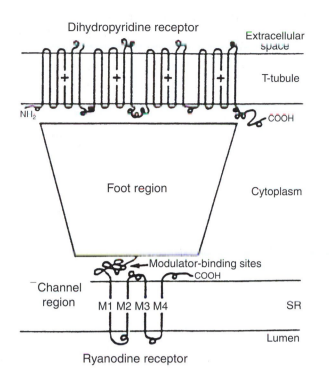

Ryanodine receptor

Figure 10.8 Schematic diagram to show the membrane topology of the ryanodine receptor in skeletal muscle. The receptor is a Ca^{2+}-release channel anchored in the sarcoplasmic reticulum (SR) membrane. Only one of its four identical subunits is shown. Each subunit is closely associated with a voltage-gated calcium channel (the dihydropyridine receptor) in the T-tubule membrane, which probably acts primarily as a voltage sensor. (From Takeshima *et al.* (1989), reprinted with permission from *Nature* **339**, copyright 1989 Macmillan Magazines Limited.)

characterized by a specific binding for the plant alkaloid ryanodine. This ryanodine receptor thus comprises a large cytoplasmic domain and an intramembrane portion. Each receptor contains four subunits, large protein chains with over 5000 amino-acid residues, so the whole complex has a molecular weight of over 2 million Da. Its intramembrane portion resides within the sarcoplasmic reticular membrane and functions as a calcium channel which in the open state would permit Ca^{2+} ions to flow out of the sarcoplasmic reticulum into the sarcoplasm surrounding the myofibrils. All the dihydropyridine receptor tetrads are closely applied to the cytoplasmic portions of such ryanodine receptors (Figure 10.8), but about half of the ryanodine receptors have no associated dihydropyridine receptors. These findings are consistent with a mechanism by which changes in the transverse tubular membrane are coupled to events in the sarcoplasmic reticulum.

10.7 | Tubular voltage detection mechanisms triggering excitation–contraction coupling

The events that couple the tubular depolarization with contractile activation likely involve detection of this voltage change by a *voltage sensor*, involving changes in molecular configuration in the tubular membrane dihydropyridine receptors. Schneider and Chandler

(1973) first detected charge movements that would reflect such a mechanism under experimental conditions designed to minimize other, ionic, currents. Imposed depolarizing steps from the resting potential to membrane voltages capable physiologically of initiating contraction then elicited an extra outward current indicating a slight non-linearity in the current–voltage curve. The current then decayed with time to a steady-state level. There was also an inward tail current that took place with the end of the test voltage steps, whose integral equalled that of the extra outward current. Furthermore, although the charge increased with increasing depolarization, the charge-membrane potential relationship was sigmoidal and saturated with large voltage displacements. These features were consistent with a charged membrane protein undergoing configurational changes within the membrane, resulting in the reversible movement of charged functional groups in response to membrane depolarization, rather than the passage of any ionic current. The currents that resulted were small in relationship to the size of ionic currents and so their occurrence would not interfere with action-potential propagation.

Currents of this kind thus result from configurational changes in the charged chemical groups that they may reflect. Such dipole relaxations would be expected to assume simple exponential decays (Adrian and Almers, 1976a,b). However, the charge movements can be separated out into a number of individual components pharmacologically and electrophysiologically (Figure 10.9). The most recognized are the q_α q_β and q_γ components. Of these, the q_β component does show such rapid exponential decays to baseline. However, it shows a voltage dependence that extends over a wide range of

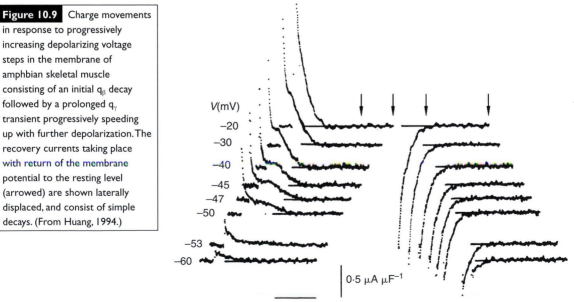

Figure 10.9 Charge movements in response to progressively increasing depolarizing voltage steps in the membrane of amphbian skeletal muscle consisting of an initial q_β decay followed by a prolonged q_γ transient progressively speeding up with further depolarization. The recovery currents taking place with return of the membrane potential to the resting level (arrowed) are shown laterally displaced, and consist of simple decays. (From Huang, 1994.)

membrane potentials reflecting a relatively gradual voltage sensitivity that would be inadequate to account for the corresponding voltage dependence of the Ca^{2+} release.

Consequently, the most interesting charge component in excitation–contraction coupling is the q_γ component. It contributes to delayed as opposed to simple exponential currents over a limited voltage range close to the contractile threshold. These can be observed independently in the absence of the earlier q_β decays under some conditions. Larger depolarizations result in these delayed components becoming larger, more rapid in time course, and merging with the earlier q_β decays. The q_γ component is thus very steeply voltage dependent, to an extent matching the corresponding dependence of the Ca^{2+} release process described in Section 10.4. It is selectively inhibited by the contractile inhibitor tetracaine, strongly suggestive of roles in the excitation–contraction coupling process. Such pharmacological properties proved useful in separating the steady-state voltage dependences of the different q_β, q_γ and q_α components of charge (Figure 10.10). The q_γ charge can persist even under conditions when sarcoplasmic reticular calcium is depleted consistent with molecular configurational changes varying steeply with membrane potential that therefore take place upstream of the Ca^{2+} release process. Following detubulation, charge movements resemble those of q_β upon which the application of tetracaine, which usually abolishes q_γ charge movement leaving q_β alone, has no impact. This localizes the q_γ charge component to the transverse tubules, whilst indicating

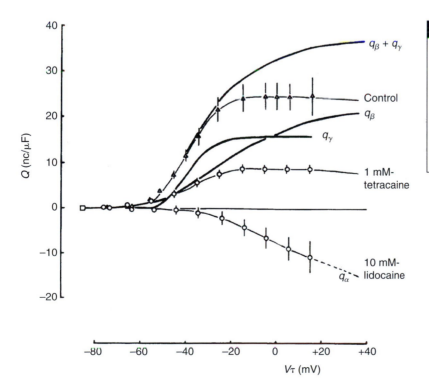

Figure 10.10 Resolution of charge–voltage curves for q_β, q_γ and q_α charge-movement components, through comparison of charge–voltage curves obtained in the absence of pharmacological agents, and following addition of the q_γ blocker tetracaine, and the q_β and q_γ blocker lidocaine. (From Huang, 1982.)

a more uniform distribution of q_β in both the surface and transverse tubular membranes (Huang and Peachey, 1989). The confinement of both the excitation–contraction coupling process and q_γ to the transverse tubules suggests that the electrical signature of the voltage sensor involved in triggering excitation–contraction coupling is likely to be q_γ.

Pharmacological studies using calcium-channel antagonists additionally identify the q_γ charge movement with configurational changes in the dihydropyridine receptor, abundant within the transverse tubules (Schwartz *et al.*, 1985), as does the parallel inhibition of sarcoplasmic reticular Ca^{2+} release by dihydropyridines (Rios and Brum, 1987). The q_γ charge is thus likely to be the electrical signature for dihydropyridine receptor action initiating excitation–contraction coupling, through which insights into the underlying configurational transitions may be derived. In direct parallel with this, nifedipine reduced the steeply voltage dependent q_γ charge movement leaving the q_β component intact (Huang, 1990). This effect showed a voltage dependence that paralleled the specific membrane binding of dihydropyridines. Furthermore the q_γ charge appeared to occur at membrane densities similar to those of the dihydropyridine receptor. Together, these findings specifically associate the q_γ both with the dihydropyridine receptor and with sensing of the transverse tubular depolarization that ultimately triggers excitation–contraction coupling. Such a sensing process may involve functional groups similar to those involved in ion-channel gating, for which the S4 voltage-sensing segment, which is rich in positive arginine residues, is of potential importance. Thus, phenylglyoxal, known to neutralize the charged groups on arginine residues, left subthreshold q_β charge intact, whilst reducing the q_γ component. This further identifies the q_γ charge with the S4 segment and, given its localization, implicates the DHPR as the excitation–contraction coupling voltage sensor.

10.8 | Calcium release from the sarcoplasmic reticulum through the ryanodine receptor

The available evidence implicates the ryanodine receptor as both the transducer of configurational change in the dihydropyridine receptor and the mediator of the resulting Ca^{2+} release. It is a large channel protein located in the sarcoplasmic reticular membrane close to the junction with the transverse tubular membrane. Genetic knockout of its expression results in a lethal dyspedia, or loss of the feet joining tubular and sarcoplasmic reticular membranes and the associated excitation–contraction coupling. Ryanodine receptor protein isolated from rabbit skeletal muscle gives rise to calcium channels blocked by either ryanodine itself, by the contractile inhibitor tetracaine, or ruthenium red, when incorporated into a lipid bilayer.

These showed properties identical to the native channels in heavy vesicles formed from the terminal cisternae of the sarcoplasmic reticulum. The gating properties of the reconstituted system were consistent with a role in excitation–contraction coupling in intact skeletal muscle. Thus both addition of ryanodine or tetracaine to the extracellular solution and ruthenium red injected into intact muscle fibres depress mechanical activity. A genetic defect in the ryanodine receptor causes *malignant hyperthermia*, an inheritable condition whose clinical manifestations of muscle spasm and excessive heat generation are typically triggered by the commonly used general anaesthetic halothane. The condition is treated by the ryanodine receptor inhibitor dantrolene sodium.

10.9 | Triggering of ryanodine receptor opening through configurational coupling to the dihydropyridine receptor

The culmination of the activation process therefore entails interactions between the dihydropyridine receptor with the ryanodine receptor. Despite their close geometrical proximity, there is little evidence for any direct electrical communication between the transverse tubules and the sarcoplasmic reticulum. Thus, the overall membrane capacitance of muscle reflects that of its surface and transverse tubules, whilst excluding that of the sarcoplasmic reticulum.

Instead, the available physiological evidence suggests a mechanical or allosteric, rather than an electrical, interaction between the two. In such a scheme, configurational changes in the dihydropyridine receptor driven by transverse tubular voltage are directly communicated to the ryanodine receptors within the sarcoplasmic reticular membrane (Figure 10.11a). Such an interaction between the two molecules in allosteric contact, opens the ryanodine receptors, thereby permitting Ca^{2+} release into the cytoplasm. The event that this coupling involves a co-operative interaction would predict a delayed charge-movement component with kinetics becoming sharply more rapid with greater depolarization, precisely as described for q_γ charge movement (Figure 10.11b).

Such a direct coupling scheme would predict that experimental modification of the ryanodine receptor, present in the sarcoplasmic reticular membrane, would reciprocally alter the properties, but not the total quantity, of the charge movement generated within the transverse tubular membrane. This was in agreement with available experimental evidence involving the specific agents summarized in Figure 10.11c. Thus, the ryanodine receptor antagonists ryanodine and daunorubicin modified the kinetics of the delayed q_γ component into monotonic decays. This action was then reversed both by the ryanodine receptor agonist caffeine, and by the lyotropic agent

Figure 10.11 Schematic representation of the functional relationship between voltage-sensing transverse tubular dihydropyridine receptors and Ca^{2+}-releasing sarcoplasmic reticular ryanodine receptors (*a*), summarizing the underlying physiological events and interactions between them (*b*) in triggering of excitation–contraction coupling. (*c*) summarizes pharmacological agents directed at either the dihydropyridine or the ryanodine receptors used in clarifying these relationships.

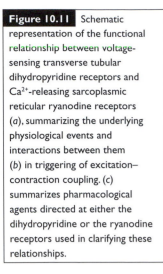
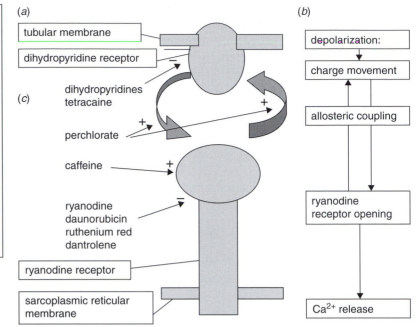

perchlorate, known to exert dissociative actions on these protein subunits. Although in cases, they shifted its dependence upon voltage, all preserved both the total quantity and the equality between net on and off q_γ charge movements (Huang, 1996). This is in contrast to the action of the dihydropyridine receptor blocking agents in actually reducing the total quantity of charge movement. However, it is consistent with actions of these agents upon a ryanodine receptor with which the dihydropyridine receptor is in direct molecular contact. Similar kinetic effects were produced by the ryanodine receptor opening agent, caffeine, which could restore a q_γ charge previously abolished by tetracaine at low, but not high, caffeine concentrations. This further suggested that ryanodine receptor opening is produced by its dissociation from the dihydropyridine receptor following transverse tubular depolarization (Huang, 1998). The resulting increase in sarcoplasmic membrane permeability to Ca^{2+} then permits an efflux of sarcoplasmic reticular Ca^{2+} into the myoplasm, whose consequently increased Ca^{2+} concentration initiates fibre contraction.

10.10 | Restoration of sarcoplasmic reticular calcium following repolarization

Repolarization restores the dihydropyridine receptors to their resting conformation, resulting in a re-setting charge movement (Figure 10.9). This would be expected to close the ryanodine receptor channels; Ca^{2+} release would then cease. However, muscle relaxation would require a re-sequestration of the released Ca²⁺ from the cytosol, and its return to its sarcoplasmic reticular store.

As indicated above, the sarcoplasmic reticulum consists of a series of membrane-bound sacs between the myofibrils. Vesicles formed from these sacs can be isolated from homogenized muscle by differential centrifugation. Their most interesting property is that they will accumulate Ca²⁺ ions against a concentration gradient. This takes place by means of a 'calcium pump' which requires energy from the splitting of ATP for its activity. The pump itself is a Ca²⁺-activated ATPase, molecular weight about 110 000 Da, which is firmly bound in the sarcoplasmic reticulum membrane. The pump serves to maintain the Ca²⁺ concentration in the sarcoplasm of the living muscle at its low resting level. It transports two Ca²⁺ ions for each molecule of ATP hydrolysed from cytosoplasm to sarcoplasmic reticular lumen, thereby restoring the resting thousandfold concentration gradient of ionized calcium across the membrane.

A number of intraluminal proteins then sequester this luminal calcium. For example, *calsequestrin* has a 1:45 binding ratio for calcium and occurs most abundantly in the terminal cisternal lumina. This sequestration process returns the cytosolic Ca²⁺ concentration to levels below those required for significant troponin binding, thereby ending the contraction.

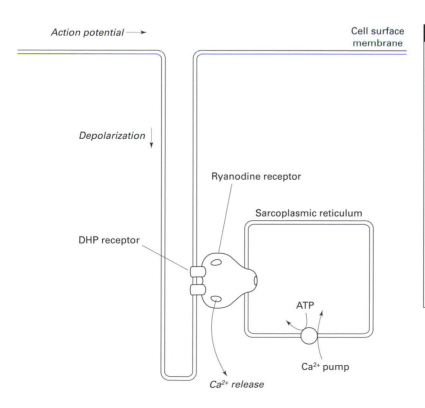

Figure 10.12 Schematic summary of the coupling process in skeletal muscle. The depolarization from the cell surface membrane spreads down the transverse tubule. The dihydropyridine receptors respond to this by opening the Ca²⁺-release channels or ryanodine receptors in the sarcoplasmic reticular membrane. Ca²⁺ ions then flow down their concentration gradient from the sarcoplasmic reticulum into the sarcoplasm, where they activate the contractile apparatus. On relaxation the Ca²⁺ ions are pumped back into the sarcoplasmic reticulum by the ATP-driven calcium pump.

10.11 | Overview of excitation–contraction coupling in skeletal muscle.

Figure 10.12 summarizes the processes recounted in this chapter. The function of skeletal muscle is to contract. This process is triggered by release of sarcoplasmic reticular calcium from the SR following surface membrane depolarization, a process known as excitation–contraction coupling. The transverse tubular system membrane is continuous with the surface membrane and so its depolarization would correspondingly result in depolarization of the transverse tubular membrane. This is detected by the dihydropyridine receptors through conformational changes that are transmitted through an allosteric coupling to the sarcoplasmic reticular ryanodine receptor. This opens the ryanodine receptor calcium-release channel. Restoration of the membrane potential re-sets the dihydropyridine receptor, and the ryanodine-receptor-mediated release of Ca^{2+} ceases. The released Ca^{2+} is then returned to the sarcoplasmic reticulum.

It is important to note that this scheme of excitation–contraction coupling varies with muscle types, although the key molecules remain the same. Thus, skeletal muscle ryanodine and dihydropyridine receptor isoforms are replaced by different specific isoforms in the heart, with implications for the fundamental mechanisms. This is considered in Chapter 12.

Contractile function in skeletal muscle

The processes described in the preceding chapters culminate in the generation of mechanical activity by skeletal muscle. These mechanical properties of muscles are readily investigated using isolated muscle or nerve–muscle preparations such as the gastrocnemius or sartorius nerve–muscle preparations in the frog. Experiments on large mammalian muscles require an intact blood supply, in which case the experiments must be performed on an anaesthetized animal, with the nerve supply to the muscle cut and its tendon dissected free and attached to some recording device. The muscle is excited by applying a brief pulse of stimulating current to its nerve or directly to the muscle itself.

11.1 | Isometric and isotonic contractions

When muscles contract they exert a force on their attachments (this force is equal to the *tension* in the muscle) and they shorten if they are permitted to do so. Hence we can measure two different variables during the contraction of a muscle: its length and its tension. Most often one of these two is maintained constant during the contraction. In *isometric* contractions the muscle is not allowed to shorten (its length is held constant) and the tension it produces is measured. In an *isotonic* contraction the load on the muscle (which is equal to the tension in the muscle) is maintained constant and its shortening is measured.

An isometric recording device has to be stiff, so that it does not in fact allow the muscle to shorten appreciably while the force is being measured. A simple method is to use a lever which is attached to a stiff spring and writes on a smoked drum. A more sophisticated device consists of a small steel bar to which semiconductor strain gauges are bonded. The electrical resistance of the strain gauges then varies with muscle tension and so can be used to give an electrical measure of the tension, and this can then be displayed on an oscilloscope or a chart recorder (Figure 11.1). The force exerted by the muscle is usually measured in Newtons or grams weight.

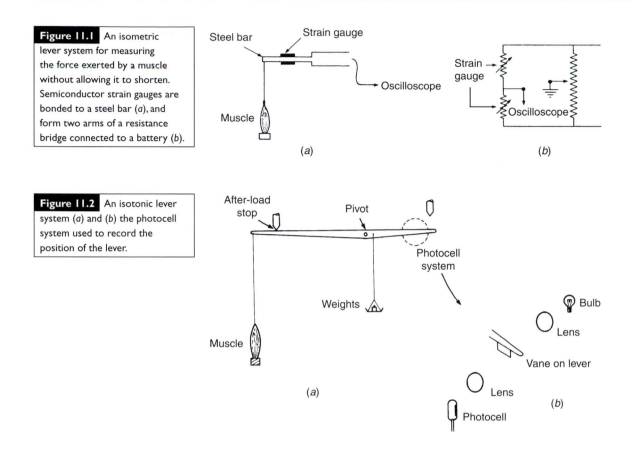

Figure 11.1 An isometric lever system for measuring the force exerted by a muscle without allowing it to shorten. Semiconductor strain gauges are bonded to a steel bar (*a*), and form two arms of a resistance bridge connected to a battery (*b*).

Figure 11.2 An isotonic lever system (*a*) and (*b*) the photocell system used to record the position of the lever.

Isotonic recording devices usually consist of a moveable lever whose motion can be recorded either directly on a smoked drum or indirectly via an electrical signal. The lever can be loaded to different extents, perhaps by hanging weights on it. Figure 11.2 shows a typical arrangement.

11.2 | Isometric twitch and tetanus

When a single high-intensity stimulus is applied to a muscle arranged for isometric recording, there is a rapid increase in tension which then decays away (Figure 11.3). This is known as a *twitch*. The duration of the twitch varies from muscle to muscle, and decreases with increasing temperature. For a frog sartorius muscle at 0 °C, a typical value for the time between the beginning of the contraction and its peak value is about 200 ms; tension falling to zero again within 800 ms.

If a second stimulus is applied before the tension in the first twitch has fallen to zero, the peak tension in the second twitch is higher than that in the first. This effect is known as *mechanical summation*. Repetitive stimulation at a low frequency thus results in a 'bumpy' tension record. As the frequency of stimulation is increased,

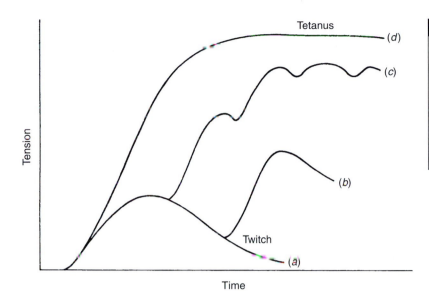

Tetanus

(d)

(c)

(b)

Twitch

(a)

Tension

Time

Figure 11.3 Isometric contractions: (a) response to a single stimulus, producing a twitch; (b) response to two stimuli, showing mechanical summation; (c) response to a train of stimuli, showing an 'unfused tetanus'; (d) response to a train of stimuli at a higher repetition rate, showing a maximal fused tetanus.

a point is reached at which the bumpiness is lost and the tension rises smoothly to reach a steady level. The muscle is then in *tetanus*, and the minimum frequency at which this occurs is known as the *fusion frequency*.

The ratio of the peak tension in an isometric twitch to the maximum tension in a tetanus is called the twitch/tetanus ratio. It may be about 0.2 for mammalian muscles at 37 °C, and rather higher for frog muscles at room temperature or below.

A low-intensity stimulus applied to the nerve may produce no contraction of the muscle; this is because the current flow is too small to excite any of the nerve fibres. As we increase the intensity of the stimulus, more and more nerve fibres are excited, so that more and more motor units are activated and hence the total tension gets greater and greater. Eventually the stimulus is of high enough intensity to excite all the nerve fibres and so all the muscle fibres are excited; further increase in stimulus intensity then does not increase the tension reached by the muscle. Thus the muscle reaches its maximum tension when all its individual muscle fibres are active simultaneously.

This mechanism provides the means by which gradation of muscular force is achieved in the body. Gentle movements involve the simultaneous activity of a small number of motor units, whereas in vigorous movements many more motor units are active.

Mammalian muscles are of two distinct types, called *fast-twitch* and *slow-twitch*. The fast-twitch muscles contract and relax more rapidly than the slow-twitch muscles, as is shown in Figure 11.4. Fast-twitch muscles are used in making fairly rapid movements, whereas the slow-twitch muscles are utilised more for the long-lasting contractions involved in the maintenance of posture. The gastrocnemius, for example, is a fast-twitch muscle used to extend the ankle

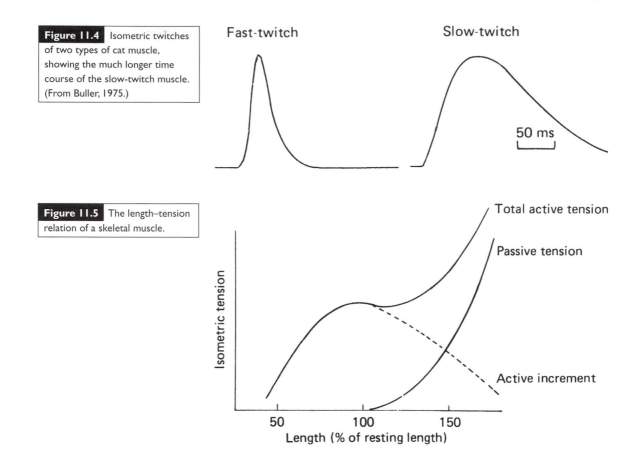

Figure 11.4 Isometric twitches of two types of cat muscle, showing the much longer time course of the slow-twitch muscle. (From Buller, 1975.)

Fast-twitch   Slow-twitch

50 ms

Figure 11.5 The length–tension relation of a skeletal muscle.

Total active tension

Passive tension

Active increment

Isometric tension

Length (% of resting length)
50   100   150

joint in walking and running, whereas the soleus is a slow-twitch muscle which acts similarly on the same joint while its owner is standing still.

When a resting muscle is stretched it becomes increasingly resistant to further extension, largely because of the connective tissue which it contains. Hence it is possible to determine a passive *length–tension curve*, as is shown in Figure 11.5. The full isometric tetanus tension of the stimulated muscle is also dependent on length, as is shown in the 'total active tension' curve in Figure 11.5. The difference between the two curves can be called the 'active increment' curve; notice that this reaches a maximum at a length near to the maximum length in the body, falling away at longer or shorter lengths, reflecting the nature of the contractile mechanism, discussed in Chapter 9 and illustrated there in Figures 9.5–9.7.

11.3 | Isotonic contractions

Figure 11.2 shows a common arrangement for recording isotonic contractions. The after-load stop serves to support the load when the muscle is relaxed and to determine the initial length of the muscle.

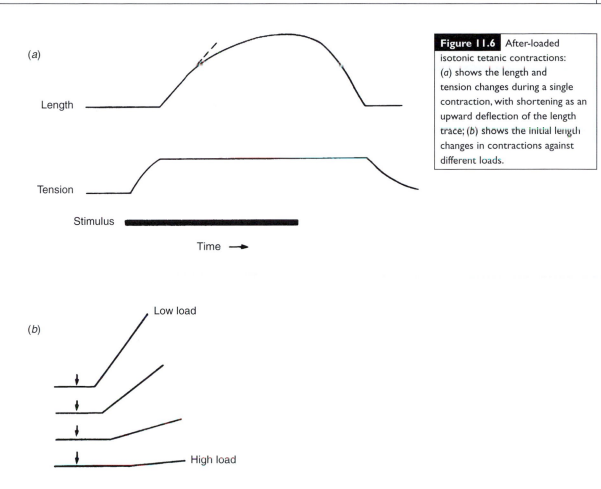

(a)

Length

Tension

Stimulus

Time ➜

Figure 11.6 After-loaded isotonic tetanic contractions: (a) shows the length and tension changes during a single contraction, with shortening as an upward deflection of the length trace; (b) shows the initial length changes in contractions against different loads.

(b)

Low load

High load

If it were not there the muscle would take up longer initial lengths with heavier loads, which would make it more difficult to interpret the results of experiments with different loads.

Figure 11.6a shows what happens when the muscle has to lift a moderate load while being stimulated tetanically. The tension in the muscle starts to rise soon after the first stimulus, but it takes some time to reach a value sufficient to lift the load, so that there is no shortening at first and the muscle is contracting isometrically. Eventually the tension becomes equal to the load and so the muscle begins to shorten; the tension remains constant during this time and the muscle contracts isotonically. It is noticeable that initially the velocity of shortening during the isotonic phase is constant, provided that the muscle was initially at a length near to its maximum length in the body. As the muscle shortens further, however, its velocity of shortening falls until eventually it can shorten no further and shortening ceases. When the period of stimulation ends, the muscle is extended by the load as it relaxes until the lever meets the after-load stop, after which relaxation becomes isometric and the tension in the muscle falls to its resting level.

Figure 11.7 Diagram showing why it is that a lightly loaded muscle can shorten further than a heavily loaded one. Starting from point *a* on the length axis, the muscle contracts isometrically until its tension is equal to the load it has to lift, and then it shortens until it meets the isometric length–tension curve. With a heavy load (*P₁*) this occurs at *x*, with a lighter load (*P₂*) it occurs at *y*. Notice that point *x* can also be reached by an isometric contraction from point *b*. (When starting from a much extended length, a muscle may in practice stop short of point *x* when lifting load *P₁*; this is probably caused by heterogeneities in muscle.).

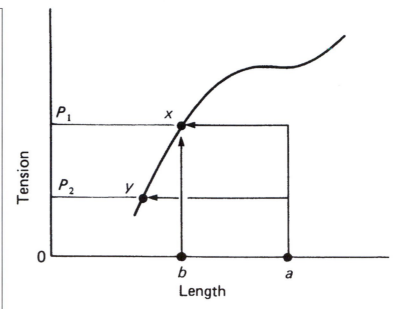

If we repeat this procedure with different loads (as in Figure 11.6*b*), we find that the contractions are affected in three ways:

(1) The delay between the stimulus and the onset of shortening is longer with heavier loads. This is because the muscle takes longer to reach the tension required to lift the load.

(2) The total amount of shortening decreases with increasing load. This is because the isometric tension falls at shorter lengths (Figure 11.5) and so the more heavily loaded muscle can only shorten by a smaller amount before its isometric tension becomes equal to the load. Figure 11.7 illustrates this point.

(3) During the constant-velocity section of the isotonic contraction, the velocity of shortening decreases with increasing load. It becomes zero when the load equals the maximum tension which can be reached during an isometric contraction of the muscle at that length.

Notice that the first two of these observations are essentially predictable from what we already know about isometric contractions. We can quantify the third observation by plotting the initial velocity of shortening against the load to give a *force–velocity curve*, as in Figure 11.8. The curve is more or less hyperbolic in shape, and is believed by many physiologists to be of fundamental importance in the understanding of muscle functioning.

In 1938, Hill produced an equation to describe the form of the force–velocity curve, as follows:

$$(P + a)(V + b) = b(P_0 - a)$$

or

$$(P + a)(V + b) = \text{constant}$$

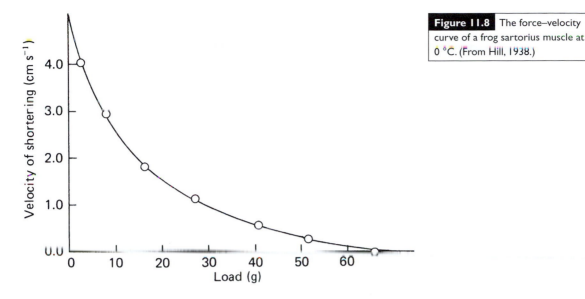

Figure 11.8 The force–velocity curve of a frog sartorius muscle at 0 °C. (From Hill, 1938.)

where V is the velocity of shortening, P is the force exerted by the muscle, P_0 is the isometric tension, and a and b are constants.

11.4 | Energetics of contraction

Energetics is the study of energy conversions. In a contracting muscle chemical energy is converted into mechanical energy (work), with heat energy being produced as a by-product. The law of the conservation of energy suggests that the chemical energy released in a contraction will be equal to the work done plus the heat given out in that contraction. That is to say,

chemical energy release = heat + work

Of the three terms in this equation, the work is the easiest to measure, then the heat, and the chemical change is the most difficult. Let us examine them in this order.

11.5 | Work and power

Mechanical energy is measured as *work* and the rate of performing work is called *power*. In an isotonic contraction, therefore, the work done is equal to the force exerted by the muscle multiplied by distance shortened, and the power output at any instant is equal to the force multiplied by the velocity of shortening.

There is no work done by the muscle as a whole during an isometric contraction since there is no shortening, and there is none done during an unloaded isotonic contraction since the force exerted is zero. Power will also be zero under both these conditions. Figure 11.9 shows how the work done in isotonic twitches (measured between

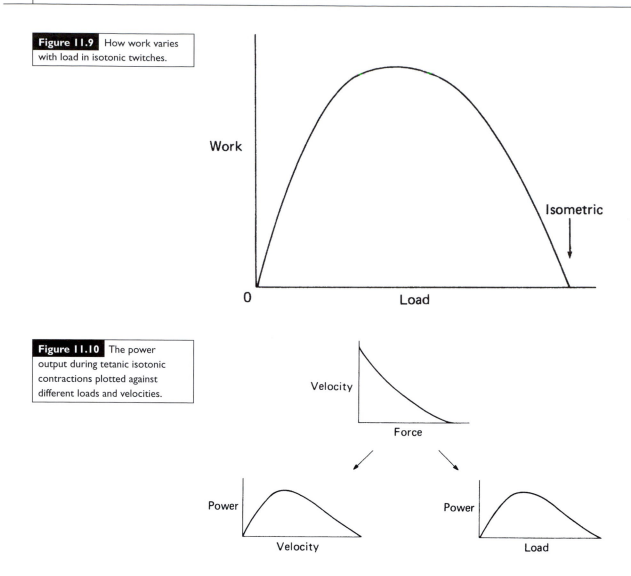

Figure 11.9 How work varies with load in isotonic twitches.

Figure 11.10 The power output during tetanic isotonic contractions plotted against different loads and velocities.

the onset of contraction and its peak) varies with the load. During the relaxation process in an isotonic twitch, the load does work on the muscle and so the overall work output during the whole of the isotonic twitch is zero.

The power output during the initial shortening phase of tetanic isotonic contractions is readily calculated from the force–velocity curve, since power is force times velocity. As shown in Figure 11.10, maximum power is achieved when the load is about 0.3 times the isometric tension, when the muscle will shorten at about 0.3 times its maximum (unloaded) velocity. This has implications for the selection of gears in cycle races: whatever the speed of the cycle, maximum power is obtained from the leg muscles when they are contracting at about 0.3 times their maximum unloaded velocity, which probably corresponds to about two revolutions of the pedals per second.

11.6 | Heat production

Our everyday experience demonstrates that muscular activity is accompanied by heat production. It is necessary to take account of this when studying the energy released by muscle. Much of our knowledge is based on that acquired by A. V. Hill and his colleagues from many years' work on isolated frog muscles. In most experiments the muscle is laid over a thermopile, an array of thermocouples arranged in series, so that very small changes in temperature can be measured.

During an isometric tetanus, heat is released at a very high rate for the first 50 ms or so (this is usually called the *activation heat*), falling rapidly to a lower more steady level which is usually called the *maintenance heat* (Figure 11.11). If the muscle is allowed to shorten, an extra amount of heat is released during the shortening process. This *heat of shortening* is roughly proportional to the distance shortened. Further heat appears during relaxation, especially if the load does work on the muscle. Finally, after relaxation, there is a prolonged *recovery heat* as the muscle metabolism restores the chemical situation in the muscle to what it was before the contraction took place.

11.7 | Efficiency

The efficiency of a muscle is a measure of the degree to which the energy expended is converted into work, i.e.

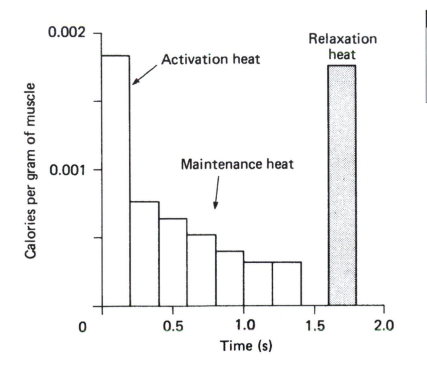

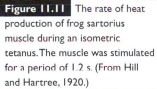

Figure 11.11 The rate of heat production of frog sartorius muscle during an isometric tetanus. The muscle was stimulated for a period of 1.2 s. (From Hill and Hartree, 1920.)

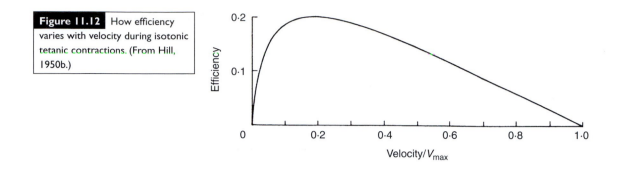

Figure 11.12 How efficiency varies with velocity during isotonic tetanic contractions. (From Hill, 1950b.)

efficiency = work/(total energy release)

= work/(heat + work)

If we consider only the energy changes during and immediately after the contraction, the efficiency works out at about 0.4 for frog muscle and 0.8 for tortoise muscle. But if we include the recovery heat in the calculation, the lower values of 0.2 and 0.35 are obtained. These are maximum values, obtained by allowing the muscle to shorten at about one-fifth of its maximum velocity. A. V. Hill's calculation of how efficiency varies with velocity of shortening is shown in Figure 11.12. Notice that maximum efficiency occurs at a lower velocity than that at which maximum power output occurs. However, both curves have fairly broad peaks so the difference between them may not be very important.

11.8 | The energy source

So far we have concentrated on the output side of the energy-balance equation. It is now time to consider the question, what chemical changes supply the energy for muscular contraction?

Energy for all bodily activities is ultimately derived from food. Food energy is transported to the muscle as glucose or fatty acids and may be stored there as glycogen (a polymer of glucose). Respiration of these substances within the muscle cells results in the production of adenosine triphosphate (ATP) from adenosine diphosphate (ADP), as is indicated in Figure 11.13. ATP appears to be the immediate source of energy for a large number of cellular activities.

The 'high-energy phosphate' can be transferred from ATP to creatine (Cr), forming creatine phosphate (CrP):

ATP + Cr → ADP + CrP

This reaction is catalyzed by the enzyme creatine phosphotransferase; it is readily reversible, so that the creatine phosphate can form a short-term 'bank' of high-energy phosphate.

This scheme is now familiar to all who study elementary biochemistry, but it is worth examining some of the evidence that it

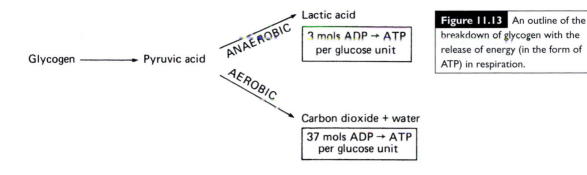

Figure 11.13 An outline of the breakdown of glycogen with the release of energy (in the form of ATP) in respiration.

applies to muscle. In 1950 A. V. Hill issued a famous 'challenge to biochemists' in which he said that if ATP really was the immediate source of chemical energy, then it should be possible to demonstrate that ATP was broken down during a contraction in living muscle.

The general method used in the experiments that followed was to use metabolic inhibitors to prevent the re-synthesis of high-energy phosphate, and then to compare its concentration in two muscles of which only one had been stimulated. The muscles had to be very rapidly frozen after the contraction (by plunging them into liquid propane, for example) so as to prevent any further biochemical change.

Davies and his colleagues (Cain *et al.*, 1962) used the substance 1-fluoro-2,4-dinitrobenzene (FDNB) to block the action of creatine phosphotransferase in frog muscles, so that ADP could not be re-phosphorylated to ATP by the breakdown of creatine phosphate. In one set of experiments they found that the stimulated muscles lost on average 0.22 µmoles of ATP per gram of muscle in an isotonic twitch. Now the heat of hydrolysis of the terminal phosphate bond of ATP is about 34 kJ/mol, so the breakdown of 0.22 µmoles should release about 7.5×10^{-3} J. The work done by the muscle amounted to 1.7×10^{-3} J per gram of muscle. This means that the ATP breakdown is more than sufficient to account for the work done in the twitch; the excess energy appears as heat.

Another way of measuring the 'fuel consumption' of the muscle is to measure the differences in creatine phosphate content of stimulated and unstimulated muscles. Here FDNB is not used because one wishes the transfer of phosphate from creatine phosphate to ATP to occur rapidly, as in the normal muscle. The re-synthesis of creatine phosphate is prevented by poisoning the muscle with iodoacetate, which blocks one of the enzymic reactions in the breakdown of glycogen, in an atmosphere of nitrogen. Under these conditions there is less creatine phosphate in the stimulated muscle than in the unstimulated one.

It has proved quite difficult to draw up a precise balance sheet for the energy changes in muscle. Wilkie (1968) made some careful measurements on the energy output (heat + work) and creatine phosphate breakdown in frog muscles during a variety of different

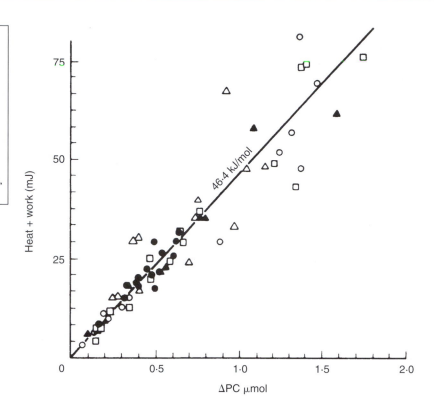

Figure 11.14 The relation between energy production (heat plus work) and creatine phosphate breakdown in frog sartorius muscles poisoned with iodoacetate and nitrogen. Each point represents a determination on one muscle after the end of a series of contractions, with different symbols for different types of contraction. (From Wilkie, 1968.)

types of contraction. His results (Figure 11.14) showed that the energy output is linearly proportional to the breakdown of creatine phosphate, with 46.4 kJ of energy being produced for each mole of creatine phosphate broken down.

However, calorific measurements suggest that the hydrolysis of creatine phosphate should yield only about 32 kJ/mol. The gap between expectation and observation became known as the 'unexplained energy'. More recent results (discussed by Homsher, 1987) suggest that at least part of this is connected with Ca^{2+}-binding reactions associated with the activation processes in the muscle, but there are still some features of muscle energy balance which are not understood.

11.9 | Muscular fatigue

The force exerted during a maximal voluntary isometric contraction in man begins to decline after a few seconds. A similar contraction in which the muscle exerts a tension of 50% of the maximum can be maintained for about a minute, and one of 15% for more than 10 minutes. This inability to maintain the tension at a particular level is called *fatigue*. It is usually accompanied by feelings of discomfort and perhaps pain in the muscle.

Experiments by Merton and his colleagues (1954) on the adductor muscle of the thumb suggest that fatigue is largely a feature of the contractile machinery of the muscle cell. The force in maximal voluntary isometric contractions declined to less than half after 1 to 3 minutes, but there was no reduction in the size of the muscle action potential produced by electrical stimulation of the motor nerve. Maximal force could not be restored by massive direct stimulation of the muscle fibres.

Fatigue has been classically related to changes in the fuel supply for the contractile machinery of the muscle. It occurs more rapidly for isometric than for isotonic contractions. Strong isometric contractions result in increased pressure within the muscle that may reduce or even completely occlude its blood supply. Consequently the muscle runs out of oxygen and hence its energy supply is soon used up. Rhythmic contractions can be maintained for a much longer time since they produce only intermittent interruptions in the blood supply.

11.10 | Energy balances during muscular exercise

The effectiveness of muscles as generators of mechanical work is thus determined in part by the speed with which they can convert their stores of chemical energy into mechanical energy. These stores may be within the muscle or outside it, and they may or may not require oxygen from outside the cell in order to be utilized. The three main energy stores are as follows:

(1) ATP and creatine phosphate in the muscle. This is the short-term energy store, amounting to about 16 kJ or so in the human body, perhaps enough for a minute of brisk walking.
(2) Glycogen in the muscle and the liver. This provides a medium-term store of very variable size: a value of 4000 kJ would not be out of the ordinary, providing enough energy for some hours of moderate exercise.
(3) Fat in the adipose tissue. This provides a long-term store: 300 000 kJ might be a typical value.

The high-energy phosphate store can be immediately utilized by the contractile apparatus of the muscle. The energy in the fat store and most of that in the glycogen store can only be utilized by aerobic respiration, for which oxygen has to be transported to the cell. The rate at which these two energy stores can be tapped is therefore limited by the rate at which oxygen can be supplied to the cell. It is for this reason that the maximum running speeds for short distances cannot be maintained over long distances (Figure 11.15).

The muscles' increased need for oxygen during steady exercise is served by the well-known physiological changes which occur in the body during exercise. The rate and depth of breathing increases, the heart rate and stroke volume increase, and the blood supply to the muscles is increased. The concentration of free fatty acids in the blood rises, as a result of the hydrolysis of some of the

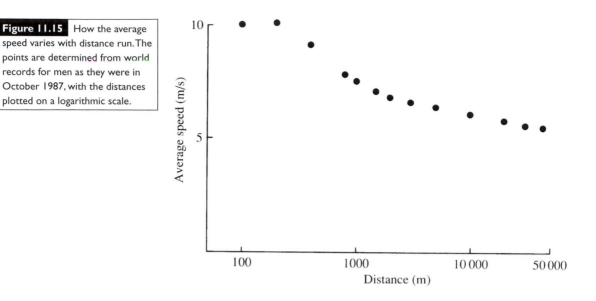

Figure 11.15 How the average speed varies with distance run. The points are determined from world records for men as they were in October 1987, with the distances plotted on a logarithmic scale.

fat stored in the adipose tissue. There is also some mobilization of the glycogen reserves of the liver.

Some of the glycogen in the muscle can contribute to the short-term energy store since it can be utilized without oxygen supplied from outside. Anaerobic respiration, producing lactic acid, supplies 3 moles of ATP per glucose unit used. This is a much less effective process than aerobic respiration, which supplies 37 moles of ATP for each glucose unit. There is also some oxygen bound to myoglobin in the muscle; this might amount to 0.41 or so, enough for a few seconds of maximal exercise.

11.11 | Ionic and osmotic balances during muscular exercise

However, sustained muscle activity also involves major shifts in electrolyte and solute balances with potential implications for its contractile function. Firstly, there are the passive inward Na^+ and outward K^+ fluxes that result from repetitive action-potential activity. These would tend to cause a loss of intracellular potassium content, but increases in extracellular K^+ concentration and intracellular sodium content. Thus, the interstitial K^+ concentration rises from the resting level of 4 mM to more than 10 mM in intensely contracting human muscle (Sejersted and Sjøgård, 2000). Such alterations in intra- and extracellular ionic concentrations would in turn tend to depolarize the cell membrane potential leading to a loss of excitability, whether of the sodium channels initiating excitation, or of the dihydropyridine receptors detecting the consequent tubular voltage changes and initiating the excitation–contraction coupling process itself.

Cellular depolarization also leads to a passive redistribution of Cl across the muscle membrane that leads to an entry of Cl⁻ and K⁺ ions. The osmotic consequence of this is a cell swelling and consequent alterations in cellular architecture that can alter transverse tubular and sarcoplasmic reticular anatomy, as well as the structure of the T-SR junctions between them coupling tubular voltage sensing to release of stored sarcoplasmic reticular calcium. It can even detach the T tubules from the surface membrane, as observed with osmotic shock of muscle (Usher-Smith et al., 2006b, 2009). For these reasons these activity-induced electrolyte shifts in active muscle have been suggested to contribute to muscle fatigue.

It appears, however, that active skeletal muscles employ a number of cellular mechanisms that counteract such depressing actions of altered intra- and extracellular ion concentrations. Thus, skeletal muscles have a high content of Na⁺-K⁺ ATPase mediating active extrusion of Na⁺ from and accumulation of K⁺ within the cells. They can increase their activity by up to 20-fold above the resting level that can take place within ~10 s of the onset of exercise and may be a limiting factor for contractile endurance. Thus, activation of the Na⁺-K⁺ pumps by β_2-agonists, calcitonin gene-related peptide, or dibutyryl cyclic 3,5-AMP restores excitability and contractile force in muscles exposed to elevated (10–12.5 mM) extracellular K⁺. Conversely, inhibition of the Na⁺, K⁺ pumps by ouabain leads to progressive loss of contractility and endurance (Clausen, 2003).

Furthermore, the membrane permeability for Cl⁻ becomes reduced by ~60% during the onset of repetitive action-potential firing in active muscle via actions of protein kinase C activation or muscle acidification (Pedersen et al., 2004, Pedersen et al., 2009). Such reduction in Cl⁻ permeability increases the excitability of muscle fibres at elevated extracellular K⁺ (Nielsen et al., 2001, Pedersen et al., 2004) and could as such counteract fatigue caused by electrolyte shift in active muscle. In contrast, with prolonged muscle activity leading to pronounced reductions in the cellular energetic state of the fibres, Cl⁻ and K⁺ permeability can suddenly increase and cause a reduction in the fibre excitability. These late elevations of the Cl⁻ and K⁺ permeabilities are particularly pronounced in fast-twitch as opposed to slow-twitch muscle and could constitute a fatiguing mechanism specific to fibre type that links cellular energetic state to the excitability of the muscle fibres (Figure 11.16) (Pedersen et al., 2009).

Secondly, anaerobic glycolysis during muscular activity results in a lactate ion accumulation resulting in intracellular concentrations up to 30 mmol/l in fast-twitch muscle, with potential osmotic effects. However, quantitative stoichiometric analysis suggests that this reflects an equimolar production of lactate and protons. Experiments in resting fibres replicating such situations demonstrated only transient volume changes following which cell volume returned to baseline. Modelling studies suggested that the final steady-state volume under these conditions depends on the relative intracellular proton-buffering power (Fraser et al., 2005) such that

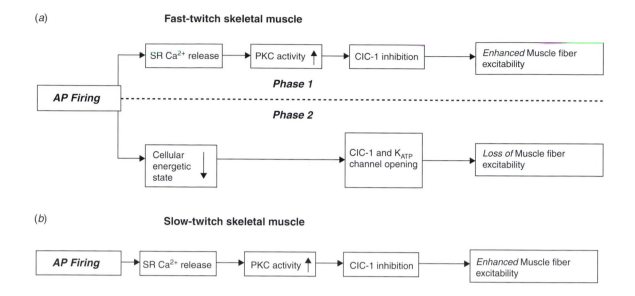

(a) **Fast-twitch skeletal muscle**

(b) **Slow-twitch skeletal muscle**

Figure 11.16 Changes in membrane conductance in relationship to their underlying cellular mechanisms during action potential (AP) firing in fast- (a) and slow-twitch (b) skeletal muscle fibres. (From Pedersen *et al.*, 2009.)

the decrease in the total charge on impermeant intracellular anions brought about by the increase in intracellular proton levels approximates the increase in lactate concentration during activity. Skeletal muscle may thus have evolved with an intracellular buffering system able to minimize any effect of anaerobic production of lactate and H+ on cell volume (Usher-Smith *et al.*, 2006a, 2009). A frequent suggestion that accumulation of intracellular lactate and hydrogen ions causes impaired function of the contractile proteins, is unlikely to be important in mammals.

Thirdly, there is a reduced Ca^{2+} sensitivity in the contractile proteins that may be partly attributed to increased levels of metabolites such as inorganic phosphate and reactive oxygen species. There is also a reduced Ca^{2+} release that might be the consequence of its precipitation as $Ca_3(PO_4)_2$ within the sarcoplasmic reticulum or an effect of reduced ATP and raised Mg^{2+} on its release process (Allen *et al.*, 2008).

11.12 | The effects of training

Muscles are markedly affected by the amount of use they receive. The structural and biochemical changes in human muscles can be investigated by the technique of needle biopsy, whereby a small piece of muscle is removed for analysis.

Muscles can be increased in size and strength by exercise involving the development of high muscle tensions, such as in isometric exercises or weightlifting. These procedures result in enlargement of the individual fibres in the muscle, including an increase in the quantity of contractile protein in them.

Training of the muscles by endurance exercises, as in distance running for example, results in an appreciable increase in the blood supply to the muscle via proliferation of the blood capillaries. The muscle fibres themselves do not increase in size very much, but there is an increase in the quantities of respiratory enzymes in them. There is also an increase in the amount of connective tissue in the muscles, so that they become less susceptible to minor injuries.

Disuse, such as occurs when a person is confined to bed or subject to prolonged weightlessness in a space station, leads to reduction of the muscle mass and especially of the contractile proteins. Hence the need for specific exercise regimes for invalids and astronauts.

Cardiac muscle

Muscle cells have become adapted to a variety of different functions during their evolution, so that in other muscle types the details of the contractile process and its control show differences from those in vertebrate skeletal muscles. These final two chapters successively examine the properties of mammalian heart and smooth muscle.

12.1 | Structure and organization of cardiac cells

Cardiac cells are considerably smaller than skeletal muscle fibres; they are typically up to 10 µm in diameter and 200 µm in length (Figure 12.1). However, adjacent cardiac cells are mechanically and electrically coupled both in a branched and in an end-to-end manner by interca- lated disks to give a syncytium through which both electrical activity and mechanical forces are transmitted (Figure 12.1a). Atrial and ven- tricular myocytes specialized to generate mechanical activity contain contractile elements whose structure is similar to that found in skel- etal muscle. Thus they also show thick myosin and thin actin filaments aligned transversely (Figure 12.1b). Cardiac myocytes are accordingly cross-striated in appearance. They similarly contain mitochondria, sarcoplasmic reticulum and transverse tubules. However, the sarcoplas- mic reticulum is less developed. In the ventricle, it makes complexes with transverse tubular membrane at *dyad* rather than triad junctions. In atrial myocytes, the transverse tubular system is considerably less developed, and sarcoplasmic reticulum makes junctions at caveolae in the membrane surface. However, there are additional cardiac cell types with differing specializations that include cells that primarily generate and conduct electrical impulses. These occur in the sino-atrial node, the atrio-ventricular node and the atrio-ventricular bundle of His. Each cell type assumes a distinct role in cardiac excitation and contraction.

12.2 | The electrical initiation of the heartbeat

Cardiac excitation thus involves an excitation of a succession of excitable and conducting structures (Figure 12.2, left). Each cardiac

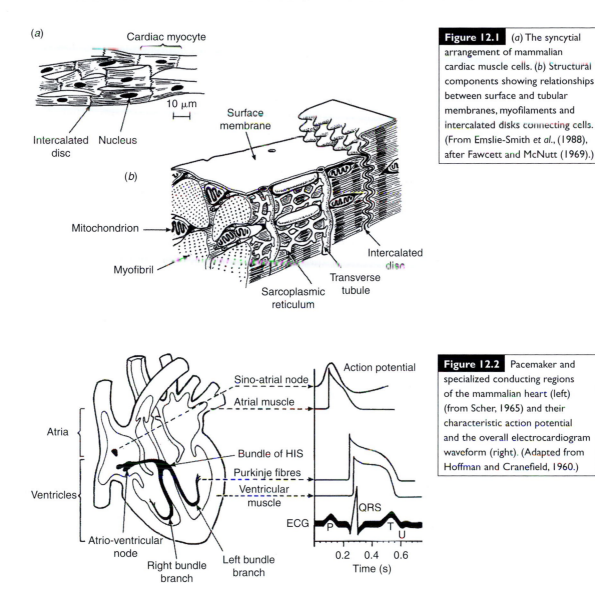

(a)

Cardiac myocyte

Intercalated disc   Nucleus

10 μm

(b)

Surface membrane

Mitochondrion

Myofibril

Sarcoplasmic reticulum

Transverse tubule

Intercalated disc

Figure 12.1 (a) The syncytial arrangement of mammalian cardiac muscle cells. (b) Structural components showing relationships between surface and tubular membranes, myofilaments and intercalated disks connecting cells. (From Emslie-Smith et al., (1988), after Fawcett and McNutt (1969).)

Atria

Ventricles

Sino-atrial node
Atrial muscle
Bundle of HIS
Purkinje fibres
Ventricular muscle

Atrio-ventricular node
Right bundle branch
Left bundle branch

Action potential

ECG

QRS
P   T
        U

0.2   0.4   0.6
Time (s)

Figure 12.2 Pacemaker and specialized conducting regions of the mammalian heart (left) (from Scher, 1965) and their characteristic action potential and the overall electrocardiogram waveform (right). (Adapted from Hoffman and Cranefield, 1960.)

cycle then results in an atrial, followed by a ventricular contraction. Cardiac activity does not require, though it is modified by, its autonomic nervous input. Its excitation process begins at the pacemaker region in the sino-atrial node, whose component cells are spontaneously active and are responsible for a rhythmic production of action potentials that determines the rate of beating of the whole heart. This pacemaker role of the sino-atrial node continues even in the absence of neural control. The sino-atrial cells then excite their neighbours by local current flow, thereby initiating a wave of depolarization across the atria. This triggers atrial contraction that forces blood into the ventricles. The atrio-ventricular ring electrically isolates the ventricles from the atria. The atrio-ventricular node provides the only communication between the two. This consists of fibres which are small in diameter resulting in a slow conduction velocity (~0.2 m/s) that ensures an appreciable delay between atrial and ventricular excitation of the atria and the ventricles. The atrio-ventricular node is connected to the large Purkinje fibres in the bundle of His. These cells show more rapid impulse propagation (~2–5 m/s) than the surrounding myocytes (~1 m/s). They thus carry the excitation on to the main mass of the ventricular muscle, beginning in the septum and then spreading from the apex of the ventricle up to its base. Purkinje cells are also potentially capable of functioning as pacemakers, but it is the cells with the highest automaticity, the sino-atrial node, that normally determine the overall heart rate. Finally, the main mass of the cardiac muscle acts as an electrical syncytium with a low electrical impedance separating the cells, permitting propagation of electrical changes from cell to cell by local current spread. This resulting pattern of activation leads to a ventricular contraction that optimizes the extrusion of blood from the chambers.

12.3 | The cardiac action potential

Cardiac action potentials were first studied through intracellular recordings from heart muscle fibres that were made using isolated bundles of canine Purkinje fibres. The Purkinje fibres form a specialized conducting system which serves to carry excitation through the ventricle. After being isolated for a short time, such fibres begin to produce rhythmic spontaneous action potentials, of the sort shown diagrammatically in Figure 12.3. The form of these action potentials differs from those of nerve axons and twitch skeletal muscle fibres in that there is a prolonged 'plateau' between the peak of the action potential and the repolarization phase. Ventricular action potentials are accordingly divided into five phases. In Purkinje fibres, a preceding slowly rising *pacemaker potential* acts as a trigger for the action potential when it crosses

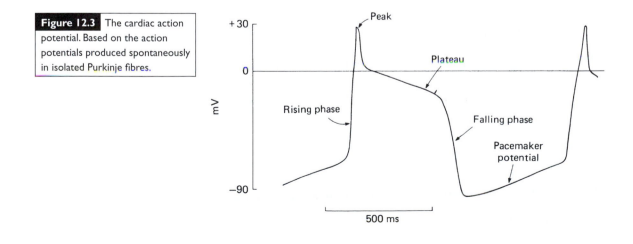

Figure 12.3 The cardiac action potential. Based on the action potentials produced spontaneously in isolated Purkinje fibres.

a threshold level. There then follows a very rapid depolarization (phase 1), an initial brief rapid repolarization (phase 2), a plateau (phase 3), a terminal repolarization that restores the membrane potential to the resting level (phase 4), which persists for a period termed electrical diastole.

Each cardiac cell type possesses particular electrophysiological properties and detailed action-potential waveforms related to their specific function (Figure 12.2, right). Sino-atrial pacemaker cells show less polarized resting potentials, marked pacemaker potentials, but an absence of the plateau phase. In both atrial and ventricular cells, the pacemaker potential is absent; in atrial cells, the plateau is replaced by a gradual sloping, triangular return to baseline, whereas ventricular cells show a prominent, sustained plateau. The long duration of the cardiac action potential as compared with that in a twitch skeletal muscle fibre is related to an important difference in their roles in excitation–contraction coupling. In skeletal muscle the action potential acts simply as a trigger which initiates the resulting contraction, but has no further control over it. But in the cardiac muscle the action potential is coincident with most of the contraction phase, and indeed relaxation begins during the repolarization phase (see Section 12.6). If the action potential is shortened in some way, relaxation begins sooner and so the tension reaches a lower peak level; the reverse happens if the action potential is lengthened. Hence the action potential acts as a controller of the contraction as well as a trigger for it.

What is the ionic basis of these heart-muscle action potentials? Sorting out the full nature of the cardiac action potential has proved to be a complicated task. In comparison with squid axons, the size and geometry of cardiac-muscle fibres makes it much harder to subject them to voltage-clamp, and the number of different ion channels involved in the action potential is larger. A computer model, based on voltage-clamp measurements on Purkinje fibres, has been produced by D. DiFrancesco and D. Noble, and serves as a useful example.

12.4 | Ionic currents in cardiac muscle

The model considers the actions of four ionic conductances. The Na^+ conductance g_{Na} is rapidly activated and then inactivated by depolarization, and blocked by tetrodotoxin though to a lesser extent than are the Na^+ conductances of nerve and skeletal muscle cells. The K^+ conductance g_K is complex, with at least three different major types of channel appearing to be involved, with some components being activated by hyperpolarization and others by depolarization. There is an appreciable Ca^{2+} conductance g_{Ca}, which is activated by depolarization and produces inward current during the plateau. A fourth conductance g_f permits the slow inward movement of Na^+

and other ions; it is activated by hyperpolarization and is important during the pacemaker potential.

12.4.1 Pacemaker activity in specialized cardiac regions

The sequence of events in the DiFrancesco–Noble model is shown in Figure 12.4. Let us begin at the point in the cycle where the membrane potential is at its most negative, at about 0.4 ms on the time trace. It has reached this negative value because the K^+ conductance g_K is high. However, the pacemaker conductance g_f has been switched on by the hyperpolarization, and it rises steadily for the next second or so. The slow Na^+ inflow which this permits results in a steady depolarization, the pacemaker potential. Pacemaker activity is important in regulating the frequency of contractile activity. Pacemaker conductances occur in the sino-atrial and atrio-ventricular nodes, in addition to Purkinje conducting tissue. Of these, under normal conditions, the high background leak conductance of sino-atrial node cells confer the highest intrinsic firing frequency of firing. This primary pacemaker accordingly determines the normal frequency of the heartbeat of around 70 min^{-1} in humans. Pathology in the sino-atrial node function as occurs in sick sinus syndrome permits the other sites with a slower intrinsic rate to act as substitute pacemakers, thereby establishing an escape rhythm. This is most frequently the atrio-ventricular node. This paces at slower (~40–60 min^{-1}) rates that nevertheless permit a normal spread of electrical activity through the Purkinje fibres into the ventricles.

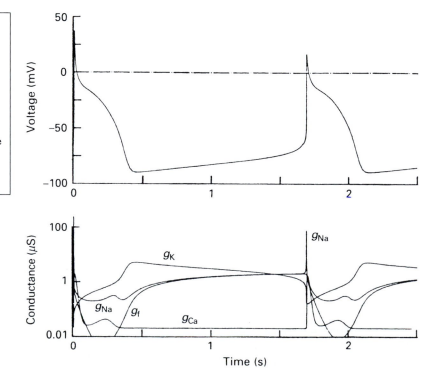

Figure 12.4 Computer simulation of the cardiac action potential. The associated conductance changes are shown in the lower graphs: g_f is the inward current which becomes apparent during the pacemaker potential. The Na^+ conductance g_{Na} includes both the conductance due to fast sodium channels and the Na^+ component of g_f. (From DiFrancesco and Noble, 1985.)

Myocardial cells whose main function is to contract are not usually able to produce pacemaker activity.

12.4.2 Phase 1 depolarization and the early rapid phase 2 repolarization driven by sodium and transient outward potassium currents

The pacemaker potential eventually drives a membrane depolarization sufficient to open the fast-activating sodium channels. This initiates the initial, rapid phase 1 depolarization brought about by a regenerative increase in the Na^+ conductance of the membrane, just as in the action potential of nerve axons. The peak membrane potential is thus reduced when the external Na^+ ion concentration is lowered. This increase in Na^+ conductance is then rapidly inactivated closing the sodium channels. Both this and activation of an early transient outward K^+ current, I_{to}, result in an early phase 2 repolarization of the membrane potential from its positive peak.

12.4.3 The phase 3 plateau phase driven by inward calcium current

In sharp contrast to the situation in nerve membrane, ventricular myocytes and Purkinje cells show a plateau phase that maintains the membrane at a depolarized potential near 0 mV for as long as 500 ms after the rapid early upstroke. This arises from a prolonged inward Ca^{2+} current initially activated by the early depolarization phase, and maintained by the sustained depolarization that results. Its amplitude varies with the extracellular Ca^{2+} concentration and is diminished by calcium-channel blockers such as verapamil and nifedipine. An inward rectifying property of the potassium channels active during this phase of the action potential results in an increased background membrane resistance. This minimizes the inward current that would otherwise be required to hold the membrane potential at the plateau level and therefore also minimizes the dissipation of Ca^{2+} concentration gradients across the cell membrane.

12.4.4 Phase 4 repolarization driven by late outward potassium currents

The repolarization phase of the action potential results from the gradual activation particularly of a further rapid I_{KR}, but also of slow I_{KS} K^+ currents to give a net outward current that drives the membrane potential back towards the resting level, and maintains it at that value, the latter ensuring a membrane-stabilizing effect, or *repolarization reserve* between action potentials. The action-potential duration appears to adjust inversely to heart rate, resulting in an adjustment of the relative durations of systole and diastole appropriate to changes in the interval between successive action potentials. Any calcium and fast sodium channels remaining open are finally closed during the repolarization phase. By the end of the action potential the pacemaker conductance g_f has already begun to rise, thus initiating a fresh cycle.

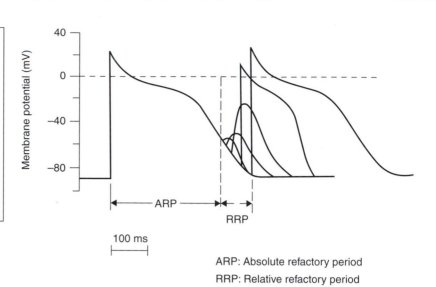

Figure 12.5 The absolute and relatively refractory periods of ventricular muscle in relationship to the action potential waveforms of ventricular muscle. Extra stimulation within the absolute refractory period results in a failure or re-excitation. Within the relatively refractory period it results in an action potential with diminished initial slope and reduced amplitude. (From Emslie-Smith et al., 1988.)

ARP: Absolute refactory period
RRP: Relative refactory period

12.4.5 The prolonged refractory period in cardiac muscle

Cardiac muscle shows a refractory period following the initial excitation that is substantially longer (up to 100 ms) than that observed in nerve. The membrane is absolutely refractory between the early rapid depolarization to the point when the membrane potential is repolarized to about −40 to −50 mV, largely owing to sodium-channel inactivation, but is relatively refractory beyond that. During the latter period the evoked action potential has a smaller amplitude, slower rate of rise and is conducted more slowly (Figure 12.5). The relatively long refractory period prevents tetany in heart muscle following repetitive stimulation, since the refractory period is long enough to allow the muscle to relax after each action potential. This is of vital importance to the functioning of the heart as a pump: the relaxation phase allows the heart to be refilled with blood from the veins before expelling it to the arteries during the contraction phase. Under normal circumstances, it also prevents premature or re-entrant excitation occurring in cardiac cells elsewhere from initiating inappropriate re-excitation and consequent arrhythmogenesis.

12.5 | The electrocardiogram

Cardiac electrical activity creates varying potentials in the body that can be recorded at skin surfaces as electrocardiograms (ECG). ECG measurement is easily performed by attaching leads to the wrists and ankles of the subject and connecting them to a suitable recording device. It is a basic investigative tool in cardiological clinical practice. Conventional ECGs were first obtained by Einthoven, using the string galvanometer which he invented for the purpose.

Their measurement is now usually performed using a hot wire pen recorder, and has long been a standard procedure in medical practice.

The ECG waveform records over time changes in potentials measured on the body surface caused by changes in the summated cardiac polarity brought about by cardiac electrical events. In the absence of such electrical polarity, the ECG would collapse to a straight isoelectric line. Deflections from this line signal the excitation processes in the heart. A positive deflection denotes an effective cardiac dipole with the positive pole facing the electrode which typically occurs when a depolarizing impulse is conducted towards the electrode or if a repolarization wave were propagating away from the electrode.

Figure 12.2 (bottom right panel) shows a typical ECG, recorded between the right arm and the left leg. The different peaks in the electrical cycle of events were labelled the P, Q, R, S and T waves by Einthoven. The events in the heart cycle to which these electrical waves correspond can be worked out by recording with surface electrodes from exposed hearts in experimental animals. Figure 12.2 (right panel) also relates different components of the ECG to waveforms resulting from electrical activity in different regions of the heart.

The P wave is produced by currents associated with the spread of excitation over the atria. The atrial re-polarization wave is either small or buried in the larger QRS complex that follows. The net currents involved in the subsequent excitation of the atrio-ventricular node and the specialized conducting tissue in the ventricle are small, because the number of cells involved is small. Their electrical activity is therefore not evident in the ECG.

The depolarization of the large mass of ventricular cells that follows is accompanied by large net currents which are seen as the QRS complex in the ECG. After this the whole of the ventricle is depolarized in the plateau phase of the action potential. There is then very little electrical current flow, resulting in a QT segment returning to the baseline. The ventricular muscle is contracting at this time to pump blood out along the aorta and pulmonary artery. Then re-polarization of the ventricular fibres occurs, at slightly different times in different places, and the current flow associated with this is seen as the T wave. After this the heart is electrically at rest except in the pacemaker regions, its muscle cells are relaxing and it is refilling with blood ready for the next cycle. Atrial pacemaker potentials preceding the next P wave reflect activity in a small number of cells and are not visible in the ECG.

The normal ECG thus conforms to a standard recognizable pattern. Deviations from this permit diagnosis of different cardiac electrophysiological disorders. Major diagnostic categories for which the ECG is useful include: (a) conduction disorders; these may range from the pacemaker cells in the SA node to the ventricular myocardium; (b) rhythm disorders, whether in the atria or ventricles and (c) metabolic disorders, whether involving electrolyte balance, or ischaemia or infarction. Any of these would result in departures from criteria for normality in an adult that include: (a) For the P wave: one before each QRS complex and ≤ 0.12 s wide and ≤ 0.3 mV high in lead II. (b) For the PR interval: consistency in length between 0.12 and ≤ 0.24 s. Shorter PR intervals suggest an existence of abnormal, accessory, conduction pathways. Longer intervals suggest first-degree heart block. (c) The QRS complex should be ≤ 0.12 s. Longer complexes can result from intraventricular conduction defect. (d) The ST segment is normally usually isoelectric. (e) The QT interval is frequency dependent, but should generally be ≤ 0.45 s. Longer QT intervals may suggest long QT syndrome.

12.6 | Cardiac excitation–contraction coupling

In common with the situation in skeletal muscle, mechanical activity in cardiac muscle is initiated by increases in cytosolic Ca^{2+} concentration following membrane depolarization. Transient rises in intracellular Ca^{2+} concentrations have thus been observed in cardiac muscle cells just as in skeletal muscle. The most important source of this activator Ca^{2+} remains its release from the sarcoplasmic reticulum following transverse tubular depolarization. Furthermore, cardiac muscle also contains specific isoforms of dihydropyridine receptors that act as voltage-gated calcium channels in the plasma membrane and ryanodine receptors that function as Ca^{2+}-release channels in the sarcoplasmic reticular membrane. However, these isoforms show detailed differences from those occuring in skeletal muscle. In consequence, the direct coupling between these receptors present in skeletal muscle does not exist in cardiac muscle. Instead Ca^{2+} currents carried by dihydropyridine receptors across the membrane surface assume central roles in cardiac-muscle activation. In addition to maintaining the plateau phase of the action potential, they produce an elevation in local cytosolic Ca^{2+} concentration. This triggers a Ca^{2+}-induced Ca^{2+} release by the ryanodine receptors. In ventricular cells, such dihydropyridine receptor activation involves a propagation of the cardiac action potential into the transverse tubules in which such receptors reside (Figure 12.6). In the smaller atrial cells, there is a much less-developed transverse tubular system. Instead dihydropyridine receptors are expressed at the cell surface. However, these come into close proximity with junctional elements of the sarcoplasmic reticulum that contain ryanodine receptors. The Ca^{2+} released by such sarcoplasmic reticular elements initiate an inward propagation of Ca^{2+}-induced Ca^{2+} release by cytoplasmic, corbular, sarcoplasmic reticulum that also contain ryanodine receptors, resulting in a centripetal wave of Ca^{2+} release beginning at the surface membrane (Figure 12.7).

These differing activation mechanisms result in increases in cytosolic Ca^{2+} concentration and tension generation that more closely track the action-potential time course than in skeletal

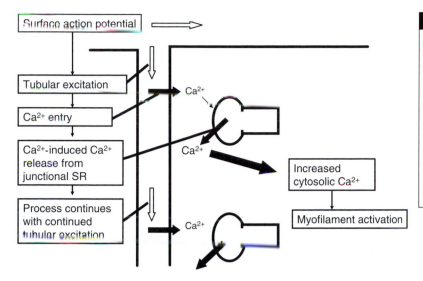

Figure 12.6 Scheme summarizing the excitation–contraction process in ventricular muscle, to be compared with Figure 10.11 for skeletal muscle. An inward wave of tubular excitation triggers Ca^{2+} currents carried by dihydropyridine receptors. This both maintains the action-potential plateau and triggers Ca^{2+}-induced Ca^{2+} release by the ryanodine receptors, thereby elevating cystolic Ca^{2+}.

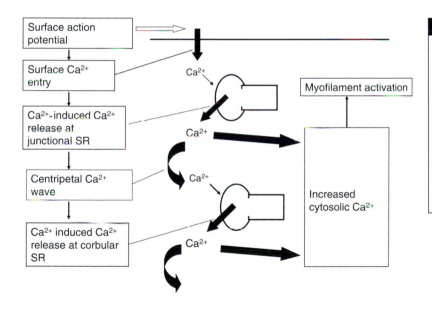

Figure 12.7 Atrial cells show less-developed transverse tubules, but express dihydropyridine receptors at the cell surface permitting Ca^{2+} entry that activates Ca^{2+} release by junctional sarcoplasmic reticular elements. This initiates an inward centripetal propagation of Ca^{2+}-induced Ca^{2+} release by cytoplasmic, corbular, sarcoplasmic reticulum that also contain ryanodine receptors, thereby elevating cystolic Ca^{2+}.

muscle, in which action-potential activation, Ca^{2+} transients and the resulting tension traces can be observed almost as sequential events (Figure 12.8). In addition, both tension generation and the cytosolic Ca^{2+} signal are profoundly influenced both by extracellular Ca^{2+} levels and factors that affect the magnitude of the inward Ca^{2+} current, as the latter would in turn ultimately influence the degree of filling of the intracellular stores. This importance of Ca^{2+} ions in heart-muscle function was first discovered by Sydney Ringer in 1883; his name has since been used to describe the saline solutions that maintain frog tissues in isolation from the body. Similarly, drugs which reduce Ca^{2+} influx reduce myocardial mechanical activity. Finally, a restoration of regular stimulation following periods

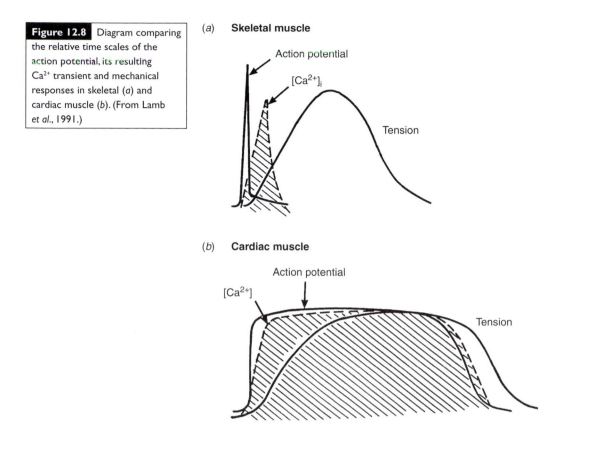

(*a*) **Skeletal muscle**

Action potential

$[Ca^{2+}]_i$

Tension

(*b*) **Cardiac muscle**

$[Ca^{2+}]$

Action potential

Tension

of cardiac quiescence that would reduce *in vitro* Ca^{2+} entry, initially results in twitches with a reduced amplitude. However, with subsequent stimulation resulting in resumption of Ca^{2+} entry, there is a successive restoration of twitch tension as stored Ca^{2+} is restored to its equilibrium levels.

An activation mechanism of this kind means that cardiac muscle also requires mechanisms that restore and maintain the intracellular cytosolic Ca^{2+} levels at their normal low concentrations following each action potential. Both surface and sarcoplasmic reticular membranes contain Ca^{2+}-ATPase pumps. These translocate Ca^{2+} ions respectively into the extracellular fluid and the sarcoplasmic reticular lumina. In addition, an Na^+–Ca^{2+} exchange system drives Ca^{2+} efflux across the surface membrane between action potentials. This utilizes the energy from the influx of Na^+ ions down an electrochemical gradient previously established by outward Na^+ and inward K^+ transport by the Na, K-ATPase. This Na^+–Ca^{2+} exchange is electrogenic: it involves an entry of three Na^+ ions for an efflux of each Ca^{2+} ion. Its increased activity following elevations in cytosolic Ca^{2+} results in a transient inward current whose depolarizing effect has been implicated in some kinds of arrhythmogenesis. Conversely, increases in intracellular Na^+ concentration decrease this inward electrochemical gradient, driving Na^+ entry and result in an increased internal Ca^{2+} concentration and contractile force. This can result following sodium pump block by digitalis and other cardiac glycosides used in the management of cardiac failure.

These cellular differences in excitation–contraction coupling mechanisms form the basis of a number of major physiological differences between the activation of cardiac and skeletal muscle. Activation of a skeletal muscle cell results in a release of a relatively constant quantity of intercellularly stored Ca^{2+} from a relatively constant sarcoplasmic reticular calcium store. This results in a relatively constant tension transient. Skeletal muscle then modulates its overall contraction strength by varying the recruitment of individual motor units and their component muscle fibres by the central nervous system. In contrast, cardiac myocytes are linked by intercalated discs into a syncytium. Each excitation therefore stimulates all muscle cells. However, intracellular Ca^{2+} release in cardiac myocytes varies with the extent of filling of their intracellular stores and a range of other intrinsic and extrinsic factors related to cardiac innervation. The overall strength of cardiac contraction is accordingly regulated by the amount of Ca^{2+} made available to the myofilaments following excitation–contraction coupling.

These properties complement further differences in the intrinsic capacity for tension generation between cardiac and skeletal muscle. Mechanical activity in cardiac muscle can similarly be studied through its tension generation during isometric contraction or through the velocity of isotonic shortening in an isolated cardiac papillary muscle subject to a constant load. This reveals length–tension relationships in resting cardiac muscle that are considerably steeper than that of skeletal muscle. This is the basis for the Frank–Starling Law of the whole heart, which states that the heart adjusts its energy of contraction in response to variations in stretch of its component muscle fibres. The heart consequently can act as a self-regulating pump that intrinsically responds to the pre-systolic filling of its cardiac chambers by returning venous blood from the peripheral circulation and which balances pumping by the right and left sides of the heart.

12.7 | Nervous control of the heart

We have seen that the heartbeat originates as repetitive activity in the cells of the pacemaker regions of the heart. This activity can be modified by the action of nerve fibres innervating the heart via the autonomic nervous system. The neurotransmitters, acetylcholine or noradrenaline, activate cellular cascades that have complex effects on cell function (Figure 8.9).

Activity in sympathetic accelerator nerve fibres increases the force and rate of the contraction. Noradrenaline is the neurotransmitter, acting on β_1-adrenergic receptors. When the noradrenaline binds to its receptor, this activates a G protein (G_s) so that the Gα subunit binds GTP and is released from the receptor and the βγ-subunit. The Gα subunit then activates the enzyme adenylyl cyclase, so producing cyclic AMP. The cyclic AMP has two effects. Firstly, it combines with open g_f channels to keep them open: this increases the pacemaker current and so increases the heart rate. Secondly, it activates protein kinase A, which then phosphorylates L-type voltage-gated calcium channels in the heart-muscle cell membrane. Phosphorylation increases the open probability of the calcium channels, so more Ca^{2+} ions enter the cell when it is next depolarized, and so the contraction force is increased.

Activity in parasympathetic inhibitor nerve fibres, on the other hand, slows the heart rate and decreases the force of the contraction. Here acetylcholine is the neurotransmitter, acting on muscarinic receptors. When the acetylcholine binds to its receptor, this activates a G protein (G_{i2}) so the Gα subunit binds GTP and splits off from the receptor and the βγ-subunit. The Gβγ subunit binds to a particular type of potassium channel (called GIRK1) and opens it, so the membrane potential is held near to E_K. There is also some inhibition of cyclic AMP production in the pacemaker cells (DiFrancesco, 1993).

Both these systems show considerable amplification. Activation of one β-adrenergic receptor activates many G proteins, each of these will activate an enzyme molecule which will produce many cyclic AMP molecules, and each activated protein kinase A molecule will phosphorylate several calcium channels. Activation of one muscarinic receptor produces many Gβγ subunits and so opens many GIRK1 channels.

12.8 | Cardiac arrhythmogenesis

The processes described above together culminate in the normal sequence of electrical activation and recovery ensuring a co-ordinated mechanical activation of the atria, and then of the ventricles. Disruptions in this normal sequence result in cardiac arrhythmogenesis. This can arise either from hereditary abnormalities or acquired clinical conditions such as hypokalaemia or acidosis. In either case, they often involve particular ion channels either decreasing net outward repolarizing currents or increasing inward depolarizing currents at particular points in the cardiac cycle. The physiological effects of such ion-channel abnormalities at the cellular level have been modelled at the level of whole hearts using murine systems that permit genetic manipulation of the expression of the ion-channel proteins involved. Murine systems have thus provided valuable models for studying fundamental arrhythmic mechanisms that might operate in a wide range of human arrhythmic conditions (see e.g. Papadatos et al., 2002).

Cardiac arrhythmogenesis can result from triggered events that arise from repeated abnormally initiated action potentials or

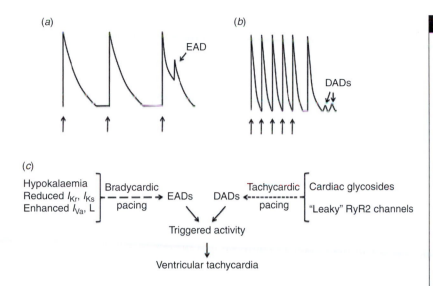

(a)

EAD

(b)

DADs

(c)

Hypokalaemia
Reduced I_{Kr}, I_{Ks}
Enhanced I_{Na}, L

Bradycardic
pacing → EADs   DADs ← Tachycardic
pacing

Cardiac glycosides
"Leaky" RyR2 channels

Triggered activity
↓
Ventricular tachycardia

extrasystoles. Alternatively, failure of excitability to recover to resting levels during or following an action potential wave can result in both *re-entrant* excitation or an arrhythmogenic *substrate* that would maintain an arrhythmic process *following* its triggering.

Triggering can result from secondary membrane depolarization occurring at the single-cell level. Early *after-depolarisations* (EADs) occur during repolarization (phases 2–3) particularly in association with action-potential prolongation (Figure 12.9) (Killeen *et al.*, 2008). The latter can provide sufficient time for re-excitation of the L-type Ca^{2+} channels normally responsible for the action-potential plateau. The resulting inward depolarizing current leads to membrane re-excitation. Such increases in action potential duration (APD) have been observed in a range of arrhythmic conditions associated with prolonged electrocardiographic QT intervals. These long QT syndromes (LQTS) are associated with increased incidences of ventricular arrhythmias and of sudden cardiac death.

In contrast, *delayed after-depolarizations* (DADs) are most frequently associated with increased sarcoplasmic reticular Ca^{2+} release mediated by the ryanodine receptor channel. This increased cytosolic Ca^{2+} results in its increased rate of expulsion by the Na^+–Ca^{2+} exchanger. However, as indicated above, this process is electrogenic and can lead to a membrane depolarization that follows full action-potential recovery. The resulting extrasystoles are thought to underlie arrhythmias observed in patients with digitalis toxicity, during sympathetic stimulation in the rare genetic condition of catecholaminergic polymorphic ventricular tachycardia associated with a range of mutations affecting the ryanodine receptor, and in heart failure.

Finally, *phase 2 re-entry* can result from retrograde propagation of an action-potential wave into regions that have recovered from refractoriness. They have been implicated in the Brugada syndrome, which in some cases is associated with an under-expression of the voltage-activated Na$^+$ channels due to their inadequate synthesis or trafficking into the cell surface membrane (Gussak and Antzelevitch, 2003)

Arrhythmogenic *substrate* maintains an arrhythmic process *following* its triggering through a slowed conduction velocity, such that each region recovers excitability before the wave returns, and uni-directional conduction block, preventing the wave from self-extinguishing. Slowed conduction can result from reduced membrane excitability or impaired intercellular coupling that increases the intracellular resistance of the pathway for action-potential propagation. It can take place with hereditary disorders resulting in an underexpression of the gap-junction protein connexin-43, acidosis and in ischaemic cardiomyopathy. Decreases in membrane excitability can take place in common conditions such as ischaemia and infarction. It can also result from the decreased Na$^+$ conductance associated with the Brugada syndrome. Uni-directional conduction block occurs under conditions permitting action-potential propagation only along a single direction, as would occur under situations in which there is heterogeneity in ventricular effective refractory period (VERP), particularly under circumstances of prolonged action-potential duration. This could result from regional differences in ion-channel expression. For example, there is a greater expression of K$^+$ currents involved in action-potential repolarization and consequently shorter APDs and VERPs in the ventricular epicardium than the endocardium (Figure 12.10).

Alterations in voltage-gated sodium channels have attracted particular interest in relationship to human cardiac arrhythmogenic conditions, and their explorations through the use of genetically

Figure 12.10 Reductions and reversals of transmural repolarization gradients in the murine heart and consequent arrhythmogenesis. Under normal conditions (solid lines), epicardial action-potential durations (APDs) are significantly smaller than the endocardial APD. Genetically modified mice with mutations in sarcolemmal ionic currents corresponding to long QT syndrome type 3 and long QT syndrome type 5 in addition to murine hearts under hypokalaemic conditions show preferential increases in epicardial compared to endocardial APD (dashed lines). These can significantly reduce or even reverse baseline transmural repolarization heterogeneities. Such effects lead to an increased incidence of spontaneous arrhythmias, in addition to arrhythmias provoked by premature extrasystolic stimuli. (From Killeen et al., 2008.)

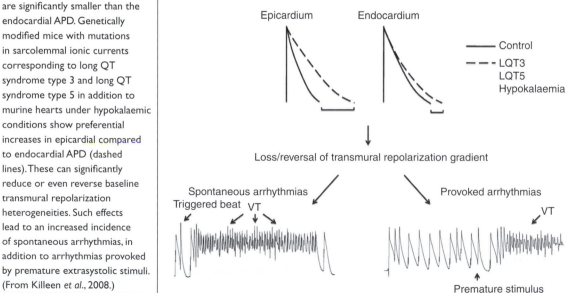

modified murine systems. Two such systems have attracted pharmacological in addition to physiological interest. They additionally usefully exemplify the contrasting consequences of mutations that result in gain- and loss-of-function genetic changes in the sodium channel. Thus, ventricular myocytes from murine Scn5a+/- hearts show a marked reduction in Na$^+$ current density (Papadatos et al., 2002) in common with the loss of sodium-channel function previously associated with some cases of the arrhythmogenic condition Brugada syndrome. They demonstrate a ventricular arrhythmic tendency that resembles the corresponding clinical features in being exacerbated by the sodium-channel blocker flecainide, but alleviated by the sodium- and potassium-channel blocker quinidine (Stokoe et al., 2007). These findings suggested an altered balance between reduced inward Na$^+$ and transient outward K$^+$ currents early in the action potential. This could permit regions of premature, phase 2 repolarization susceptible to re-entrant excitation. The loss of sodium-channel function would also account for alterations in atrial pacemaking and conduction function in the same hearts (Lei et al., 2005). Conversely, murine hearts with the gain-of-function mutation Scn5a+/ΔKPQ, show deletion of three conserved amino acids in the sodium channel, clinically associated with long QT syndrome type 3. These show evidence for prolonged epicardial action-potential durations owing to compromised sodium-channel inactivation, that alter transventricular repolarization gradients in the opposite direction, thereby offering a contrasting arrhythmogenic mechanism. Flecainide now alleviates, but quinidine exacerbates arrhythmogenesis, fulfilling expectations from the known effects of flecainide and quinidine in inhibiting inward Na$^+$ and transient outward currents responsible for action-potential depolarization and re-polarization, respectively.

Smooth muscle

Smooth, unstriated muscle forms the muscular component in the walls of hollow organs such as the gastrointestinal tract, the trachea, bronchi and bronchioles of the respiratory system, blood vessels in the cardiovascular system and the urogenital system. Smooth muscle contracts and relaxes much more slowly than skeletal muscle, but is much better adapted to sustained contractions. The load against which smooth muscle works is typically the pressure within the tubular structures that they line. In organs such as the blood vessels, they are responsible for a steady intraluminal pressure brought about by their tonic contraction. In the gastrointestinal tract, they produce a phasic contraction that propels its contents onward. They also occur in the iris, ciliary body and nictitating membrane in the eye, and are the small muscles which erect the hairs. The functions of smooth muscle in the body are thus diverse. This is reflected in their wide variations in structure and detailed physiological properties, for which this chapter only provides a brief introduction.

13.1 | Structure

Smooth muscle cells (Figure 13.1) are uni-nucleate, elongated, often spindle-shaped and much smaller than the multi-nucleate skeletal muscle fibres. They are typically 3–5 µm in diameter and up to 400 µm long. Their thick myosin and thin actin filaments are arranged longitudinally in the cytoplasm, but are not aligned transversely. The cells consequently show no visible striations or sarcomeres. The actin filaments are attached in bundles at *dense bodies* in the cytoplasm, and to *attachment plaques* at the membrane. The latter are analogous to the Z disks in skeletal muscle and also contain α-actinin. These act as anchors for filaments to permit effective cell shortening. There is a vesicular sarcoplasmic reticulum close to the membrane, but no T tubular system. Adjacent cells are connected at regions where the opposing cell membranes are brought close together to form gap junctions. These likely allow propagation of waves of electrical excitation or intracellular messengers through the tissue.

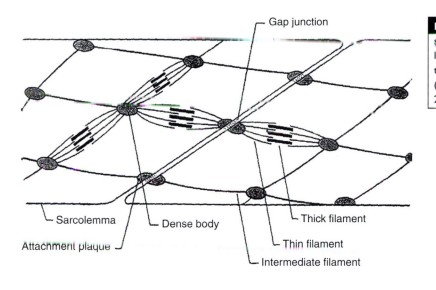

Gap junction

Sarcolemma — Dense body — Thick filament

Attachment plaque — Thin filament — Intermediate filament

Figure 13.1 Basic features of smooth muscle cells showing layout of gap junctions, thick and thin filaments, and dense bodies. (From Koeppen and Stanton, 2009.)

13.2 | Excitation

Smooth muscle receives both hormonal and autonomic, involuntary, nervous regulatory input. The latter often takes the form of a reciprocal innervation by both sympathetic and parasympathetic fibres that form loosely associated terminals on the membrane surface. Their released transmitter diffuses and acts over a wide area of the muscle. However, in contrast to skeletal muscle, smooth muscle can generate active tension in the absence of nerve activity: neuronal input often simply *modulates* rather than initiates smooth-muscle tension.

Many smooth muscles thus show a great deal of spontaneous activity. This is particularly so in intestinal muscles, where spontaneous contractions mix and propel the gut contents. Their electrical activity consists of slow waves of variable amplitude and all-or-nothing action potentials (Figure 13.2). The fibres are depolarized and the frequency of action potentials increases if the muscle is stretched. The spontaneous activity can be modified by the action of extrinsic nerves, by adrenaline, and in uterine muscle by the action of hormones of the reproductive cycle. Smooth muscles of the iris, nictitating membrane and vas deferens are not spontaneously active.

The action potentials last for several milliseconds and are thus much longer than those of nerve axons and skeletal muscle cells. They are insensitive to tetrodotoxin and can often be produced in the absence of Na^+ ions, but are prevented by calcium-channel blocking agents such as nifedipine. This suggests that Ca^{2+} ions are the main carriers of inward current. Action potentials can be initiated in sheets or strips of smooth muscle by electrical stimulation; they will then propagate along the axes of the muscle cells from

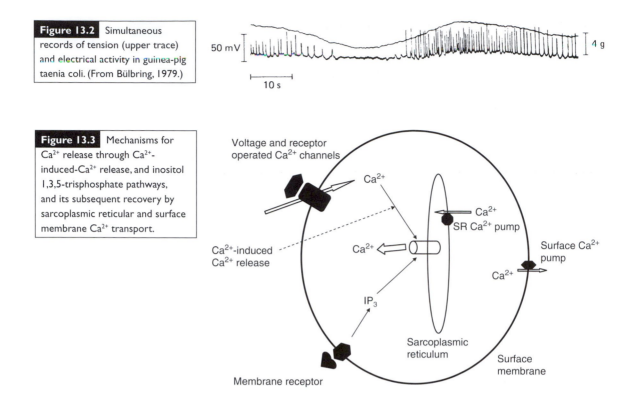

Figure 13.2 Simultaneous records of tension (upper trace) and electrical activity in guinea-pig taenia coli. (From Bülbring, 1979.)

50 mV

10 s

4 g

Figure 13.3 Mechanisms for Ca²⁺ release through Ca²⁺-induced-Ca²⁺ release, and inositol 1,3,5-trisphosphate pathways, and its subsequent recovery by sarcoplasmic reticular and surface membrane Ca²⁺ transport.

Voltage and receptor operated Ca²⁺ channels

Ca²⁺

Ca²⁺
SR Ca²⁺ pump

Ca²⁺-induced Ca²⁺ release

Ca²⁺

Surface Ca²⁺ pump

Ca²⁺

IP₃

Sarcoplasmic reticulum

Surface membrane

Membrane receptor

one cell to another. There is also some slower propagation across the axes of the cells. The electrical changes produced by nervous action on these cells spread to nearby cells by current flow from cell to cell, probably through the gap junctions by which they are connected. Stimulation of the nerves results in post-synaptic potentials of various types. Excitatory nerves produce depolarizing potentials, whereas inhibitory nerves produce hyperpolarizing ones.

There are a number of transmitter substances involved. Acetylcholine, acting on muscarinic receptors, is an excitatory transmitter in much intestinal muscle and in the iris. Noradrenaline is excitatory at some sites, as in the vas deferens, and inhibitory at others, as in intestinal muscle and the iris of the eye. Other neurotransmitters are active at various sites: candidates include ATP, nitric oxide and various peptides such as substance P, vasointestinal peptide (VIP) and others.

13.3 | Excitation–contraction coupling

As in other muscle types, Ca²⁺ ions trigger excitation–contraction coupling (Figure 13.3). Depolarization opens calcium channels, allowing Ca²⁺ to enter the cell. These may in turn release further Ca²⁺ by activating Ca²⁺-release channels in the sarcoplasmic reticulum. An alternative route for Ca²⁺ release is via the production of inositol-1,4,5-trisphosphate (IP_3) through the action of membrane-associated phospholipase C (PLC), upon membrane phosphoinositide lipid (PIP_2). This follows activation of G-protein-coupled 7TM receptors. The IP_3 combines with IP_3 receptors in the sarcoplasmic reticular membrane and these in turn release Ca^{2+} ions into the cytoplasm. In addition to voltage-gated calcium channels, there are several other sources of intracellular Ca^{2+} elevation. Receptor-operated Ca^{2+}-permeable channels activated by hormones or neurotransmitters can also mediate Ca^{2+} influx, without prior depolarization. Following activity, intracellular free Ca^{2+} levels are reduced to their low resting levels by ATP-utilizing Ca^{2+} pumps in the plasma membrane and in the sarcoplasmic reticulum, thus replenishing the latter's Ca^{2+} store.

13.4 | Contractile mechanism

Smooth muscles contain the major contractile proteins actin and myosin, together with tropomyosin, with a lower relative proportion of myosin than in skeletal muscles. In contrast to the situation in skeletal muscle, the myosin molecules within the thick filaments are oriented in opposite directions on the two faces of a filament. This permits a thin filament to be pulled over the whole of its length by a thick filament, so that the muscle can operate at near maximum tension over a wide range of lengths (Figure 13.4).

Contractile activation is similarly more complex and subject to modulation. It involves a range of biochemical cascades that account for the considerably slower kinetics of mechanical activation. Crossbridge activity is controlled by a range of different mechanisms. Although all depend on increases in cytosolic Ca^{2+}, they involve its initial combination with calmodulin rather than actions involving troponin. The latter is absent in smooth muscle.

At the level of the actin filaments, the calcium–calmodulin complex binds to the protein caldesmon resulting in its dissociation from the actin–tropomyosin thin filaments thereby permitting their interaction with myosin, and consequent crossbridge cycling (Figure 13.5a). Such a dissociation of caldesmon can also directly result from its phosphorylation by protein kinase C (PKC), in turn activated by diacylglycerol (DAG), another product of phospholipase C activation (Figure 13.5b).

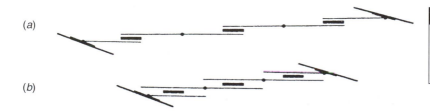

(a)

(b)

Figure 13.4 A contractile unit of smooth muscle, showing how the filaments could slide past each other during contraction. (From Squire, 1986.)

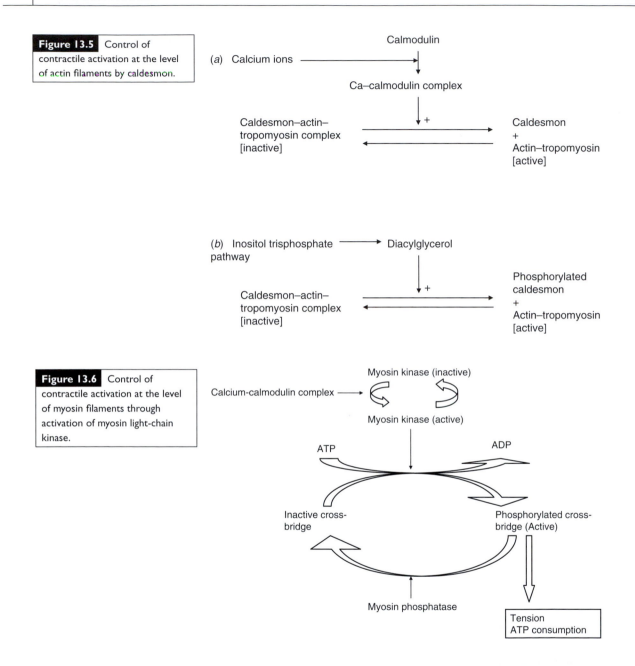

Figure 13.5 Control of contractile activation at the level of actin filaments by caldesmon.

(a) Calcium ions ⟶ Calmodulin ⟶ Ca–calmodulin complex

Caldesmon–actin–tropomyosin complex [inactive] ⇌ (+) Caldesmon + Actin–tropomyosin [active]

(b) Inositol trisphosphate pathway ⟶ Diacylglycerol

Caldesmon–actin–tropomyosin complex [inactive] ⇌ (+) Phosphorylated caldesmon + Actin–tropomyosin [active]

Figure 13.6 Control of contractile activation at the level of myosin filaments through activation of myosin light-chain kinase.

Calcium-calmodulin complex ⟶ Myosin kinase (inactive) / Myosin kinase (active)

ATP / ADP

Inactive cross-bridge

Phosphorylated cross-bridge (Active)

Myosin phosphatase

Tension ATP consumption

At the level of the myosin filaments, the calcium–calmodulin complex activates the enzyme myosin light-chain kinase. This in turn catalyses phosphorylation of the myosin light chain MLC_{20}. This phosphorylation involves formation of a covalent bond and therefore constitutes a form of covalent regulation. This initiates cross-bridge cycling and its associated splitting of ATP (Figure 13.6). Direct Ca^{2+} binding to the myosin light chain also increases crossbridge cycling.

The cross-bridge cycling ceases when the light chain is dephosphorylated by myosin phosphatase. Dephosphorylation at a stage

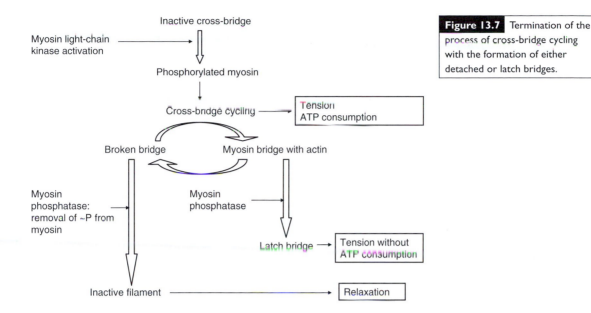

Figure 13.7 Termination of the process of cross-bridge cycling with the formation of either detached or latch bridges.

when the myosin and the thin filament are detached permits muscle relaxation and an end of contractile activity (Figure 13.7). In contrast, if dephosphorylation occurs when the myosin is attached to the thin filament, it then remains bound with high affinity. Cross-bridges in this state are termed latch bridges. They allow a maintained tension without a requirement for cross-bridge cycling or ATP consumption. This mechanism explains the greater ~300-fold energy efficiency of smooth compared to skeletal muscle during maintained contractions. The cellular levels of the kinases and phosphatase involved in this regulation can be modulated to make long-term adjustments to the contractile properties of smooth muscle cells.

13.5 | Mechanical properties

Isometric contraction in smooth muscle shows a force–length relationship that resembles that of skeletal muscle, implicating a similar, fundamental, sliding-filament mechanism, despite its lack of obvious sarcomere structure. Maximal contraction velocity is much lower than in skeletal muscle, but continues to show an inverse, Hill, relationship to load during isotonic contractions. In addition, shortening velocity in smooth muscle can be increased by increasing the levels of cross-bridge phosphorylation. However, a near maximal isometric *force*, can be generated even at low phosphorylation levels. In a maintained contraction, therefore, Ca^{2+} and the rate of cross-bridge phosphorylation first rise to their peak levels, to produce rapid shortening, and then subside to much lower levels, while tension is maintained.

Many smooth muscles, such as those in bladder, uterus and gut, contract phasically in response to stretch. This is the result of mechanically induced depolarization, brought about by stretch-activated intramembrane ion channels. This plays a rôle in peristaltic movements in the intestine. Other smooth muscles show a tonic stretch-induced contraction that allows compensatory adjustment of tension. A constant muscle fibre length gets consequently maintained despite variations in load, as occurs in the response of arteriolar smooth muscle to raised blood pressure.

Further reading

Adrian, R. H. and Peachey, L. D. (1983). Skeletal muscle. *Handbook of Physiology*, Section 10. Bethesda, MD: American Physiological Society.

Aidley, D. J. (1998). *The Physiology of Excitable Cells*, 4th edn. Cambridge: Cambridge University Press.

Aidley, D. J. and Stanfield, P. R. (1996). *Ion Channels: Molecules in Action*. Cambridge: Cambridge University Press.

Bagshaw, C. R. (1993). *Muscle Contraction*, 2nd edn. London: Chapman & Hall.

Bers, D. M. (1991). *Excitation Contraction Coupling and Cardiac Contractile Force*. Dordrecht: Kluwer.

Brown, H. and Kozlowski, R. (1997). *Physiology and Pharmacology of the Heart*. Oxford. WileyBlackwell.

Gussak, I. and Antzelevich, C. (2003). *Cardiac Repolarization: Bridging Basic and Clinical Science*. Totowa, NJ: Humana Press, Inc.

Hille, B. (2001). *Ionic Channels of Excitable Membranes*, 3rd edn. Sunderland, Massachusetts: Sinauer Associates.

Hodgkin, A. L. (1992). *Chance and Design*. Cambridge: Cambridge University Press.

Huang, C. L-H. (1994). *Intramembrane Charge Movements in Striated Muscle*. Oxford: Oxford University Press.

Kao, C. Y. and Carsten, M. E. (2005). *Cellular Aspects of Smooth Muscle Function*. Cambridge: Cambridge University Press.

Keynes, R. D. (1994). The kinetics of voltage-gated ion channels. *Q. Rev. Biophys.* **27**, 339–434.

Koeppen, B. M. and Stanton, B. A. (2009). *Berne & Levy: Principles of Physiology*, 6th edn. New York: Mosby, 848pp.

Lei, M., Grace, A. A. and Huang, C. L-H. (eds.) (2008). Double focus issue: Translational models for cardiac arrhythmogenesis. *Prog. in Biophys. Molec. Biol.* **98** [ed. D. Noble and T. Blundell]. Theme double issue.

Nicholls, C. G., Fuchs, P. A., Martin, A. R. and Wallace, B (2001). *From Neuron to Brain: Cellular Approach to the Function of the Nervous System*, 3rd edn. Sunderland, MA: Sinauer Associates Inc.

Noble, D. (1984). *The Initiation of the Heartbeat*, 3rd edn. Oxford: Oxford University Press.

Noble, D. (2008). *The Music of Life: Biology Beyond Genes*. Oxford: Oxford University Press.

Sugi, H. (2004). *Molecular and Cellular Aspects of Muscle Contraction* (*Advances in Experimental Medicine and Biology*). New York: Springer.

Zipes, D. P. and Jalife, J. (2004). *Cardiac Electrophysiology: From Cell to Bedside*. 4th edn. Philadelphia, PA: Saunders.

References

Adrian, E. D. and Lucas, K. (1912). On the summation of propagated disturbances in nerve and muscle. *J. Physiol., Lond.* **44**, 68–124.

Adrian, R.H. and Almers, W. (1976a). The voltage dependence of membrane capacity. *J. Physiol., Lond.* **254**, 317–338.

Adrian, R.H. and Almers, W. (1976b). Charge movement in the membrane of striated muscle. *J. Physiol., Lond.* **254**, 339–360.

Adrian, R. H. and Bryant, S. H. (1974). On the repetitive discharge in myotonic muscle fibres. *J. Physiol.* **240**, 505–515.

Adrian, R. H. and Peachey, L.D. (1973). Reconstruction of the action potential of frog sartorius muscle. *J. Physiol.* **235**, 103–131.

Ahern, C. A. and Horn, R. (2005). Focused electric field across the voltage sensor of potassium channels. *Neuron* **48**, 25–29.

Aidley, D. J. (1998). *The Physiology of Excitable Cells*, 4th edn. Cambridge: Cambridge University Press.

Allen, D. G., Lamb, G. D. and Westerblad, H. (2008). Skeletal muscle fatigue: cellular mechanisms. *Physiol. Rev.* **88**, 287–332.

Armstrong, C. M. and Bezanilla, F. M. (1973). Current related to the movement of the gating particle of the sodium channels. *Nature* **242**, 459–461.

Ashley, C. C. and Ridgeway, E. B. (1968). Simultaneous recording of membrane potential, calcium transient and tension in single muscle fibres. *Nature* **219**, 1168–1169.

Bagshaw, C. R. (1993). *Muscle Contraction*, 2nd edn. London: Chapman & Hall.

Baker, P. F., Hodgkin, A. L. and Shaw, T. I. (1962). The effect of changes in internal ionic concentrations on the electrical properties of perfused giant axons. *J. Physiol.* **164**, 355–374.

Barnard, E. A., Miledi, R. and Sumikawa, K. (1982). Translation of exogenous messenger RNA coding for nicotinic acetylcholine receptors produces functional receptors in Xenopus oocytes. *Proc. R. Soc. Lond.* **B215**, 241–246.

Block, B. A., Imagawa, T., Campbell, K. P. and Franzini-Armstrong, C. (1988). Structural evidence for direct interaction between the molecular components of the transverse tubule/sarcoplasmic reticulum junction in skeletal muscle. *J. Cell Biol.* **107**, 2587–2600.

Boyle, P. J. and Conway, E. J. (1941). Potassium accumulation in muscle and associated changes. *J. Physiol.* **100**, 1–63.

Brock, L. G., Coombs, J. S. and Eccles, J. C. (1952). The recording of potentials from motoneurones with an intracellular electrode. *J. Physiol.* **117**, 431–460.

Broomand, A. and Elinder, F. (2008). Large-scale movement within the voltage-sensor paddle of a potassium channel-support for a helical-screw motion. *Neuron* **59**, 770–777.

Bülbring, E. (1979). Post junctional adrenergic mechanisms. *Brit. Med. Bull.* **35**, 285–294.

Buller, A. J. (1975). *The Contractile Behaviour of Mammalian Skeletal Muscle* (Oxford Biology Reader No. 36). London: Oxford University Press.

Cain, D. F., Infante, A. A. and Davies, R. E. (1962). Chemistry of muscle contraction. Adenosine triphosphate and phosphoryl creatine as energy supplies for single contractions of working muscle. *Nature* **196**, 214–217.

Caldwell, P. C., Hodgkin, A. L., Keynes, R. D. and Shaw, T. I. (1960). The effects of injecting 'energy-rich' phosphate compounds on the active transport of ions in the giant axons of *Loligo*. *J. Physiol.* **152**, 561–590.

Caldwell, P. C. and Keynes, R. D. (1957). The utilization of phosphate bond energy for sodium extrusion from giant axons. *J. Physiol.* **137**, 12–13P.

Catterall, W. A. (1986). Molecular properties of voltage-sensitive sodium channels. *Ann. Rev. Biochem.* **55**, 953–985.

Catterall, W. A. (1992). Cellular and molecular biology of voltage-gated ion channels. *Physiol. Rev.* **72**, S15–S48.

Catterall, W. A. (2001). A one-domain voltage-gated sodium channel in bacteria. *Science* **294**, 2306–2308.

Chandler, W. K. and Meves, H. (1970). Evidence for two types of sodium conductance in axons perfused with sodium fluoride solution. *J. Physiol.* **211**, 653–678.

Clausen, T. (2003) Na+-K+ pump regulation and skeletal muscle contractility. *Physiol. Rev.* **83**, 1269–1324.

Cole, K. S. and Curtis, H. J. (1939). Electric impedance of the squid giant axon during activity. *J. Gen. Physiol.* **22**, 649–670.

Colquhoun, D. and Sakmann, B. (1985). Fast events in single-channel currents activated by acetylcholine and its analogues at the frog muscle end-plate. *J. Physiol.* **369**, 501–557.

Conway, E. J. (1957). Nature and significance of concentration relations of potassium and sodium ions in skeletal muscle. *Physiol. Rev.* **37**, 84–132.

Coombs, J. S., Eccles, J. C. and Fatt, P. (1955a). Excitatory synaptic action in motoneurones. *J. Physiol.* **130**, 374–395.

Coombs, J. S., Eccles, J. C. and Fatt, P. (1955b). The specific ionic conductances and the ionic movements across the motoneuronal membrane that produce the inhibitory postsynaptic potential. *J. Physiol.* **130**, 326–373.

Dale, H. H., Feldburg, W. and Vogt, M. (1936). Release of acetylcholine at voluntary motor nerve endings. *J. Physiol.* **86**, 353–380.

Davson, H. and Danielli, J. F. (1943). *The Permeability of Natural Membranes.* Cambridge: Cambridge University Press.

del Castillo, J. and Katz, B. (1954). Quantal components of the end-plate potential. *J. Physiol.* **124**, 560–573.

del Castillo, J. and Katz, B. (1955). On the localization of acetylcholine receptors. *J. Physiol.* **128**, 157–181.

del Castillo, J. and Moore, J. W. (1959). On increasing the velocity of a nerve impulse. *J. Physiol.* **148**, 665–670.

diFrancesco, D. (1993). Pacemaker mechanisms in cardiac tissue. *Ann. Rev. Physiol.* **55**, 455–472.

diFrancesco, D. and Noble D. (1985). A model of cardiac electrical activity incorporating ionic pumps and concentration changes. *Phil. Trans. R. Soc. Lond.* **B307**, 353–398.

Doyle, D. A., Cabral, J. M., Pfuetzen, R. A. *et al.* (1998). The structure of the potassium channel: molecular basis of K+ conduction and selectivity. *Science* **280**, 69–77.

Eccles, J. C. (1964). *The Physiology of Synapses.* Berlin: Springer Verlag.

Einthoven, W. (1924). The string galvanometer and measurement of the action currents of the heart. Nobel Lecture. Republished in 1965 in *Nobel Lectures, Physiology or Medicine 1921–41.* Amsterdam: Elsevier.

Emslie-Smith, D., Paterson C.R., Scratcherd T. and Read N.W. (1988). *Textbook of Physiology,* 11th edn. Edinburgh: Churchill-Livingstone.

Erlanger, J. and Gasser, H. S. (1937). *Electrical Signs of Nervous Activity*. Philadelphia: University of Pennsylvania Press.

Fatt, P. and Katz, B. (1951). An analysis of the end-plate potential recorded with an intracellular electrode. *J. Physiol.* **115**, 320–369.

Fatt, P. and Katz, B. (1952). Spontaneous subthreshold activity at motor nerve endings. *J. Physiol.* **117**, 109–128.

Fawcett, D.W. and McNutt, N. S. (1969). The ultrastructure of cat myocardium. I. Ventricular papillary muscle. *J. Cell Biol.* **42**, 1–45.

Ferenczi, E. A., Fraser, J. A., Chawla, S. *et al.* (2004). Membrane potential stabilization in amphibian skeletal muscle fibres in hypertonic solutions. *J. Physiol.* **555**, 423–438.

Frankenhaeuser, B. and Hodgkin, A. L. (1957). The action of calcium on the electrical properties of squid axons. *J. Physiol.* **137**, 218–244.

Franzini-Armstrong, C. and Jorgensen, A. O. (1994). Structure and development of e–c coupling units in skeletal muscle. *Ann. Rev. Physiol.* **56**, 509–534.

Fraser, J. A. and Huang, C. L.-H. (2004). A quantitative analysis of cell volume and resting potential determination and regulation in excitable cells. *J. Physiol.* **559**, 459–478.

Fraser, J. A. and Huang, C. L.-H. (2007). Quantitative techniques for steady-state calculation and dynamic integrated modelling of membrane potential and intracellular ion concentrations. *Prog. Biophys. Mol. Biol.* **94**, 336–372.

Fraser, J. A., Middlebrook, C. E., Usher-Smith, J. A., Schweining, C. J. and Huang, C. L.-H. (2005). The effect of intracellular acidification on the relationship between cell volume and membrane potential in amphibian skeletal muscle. *J. Physiol.* **563**, 745–764.

Fraser, J. A., Skepper, J. N., Hockaday, A. R. and Huang, C. L.-H. (1998). The tubular vacuolation process in amphibian skeletal muscle. *J. Musc. Res. Cell Motility* **19**, 613–629.

Gordon, A. M., Huxley, A. F. and Julian, F. J. (1966). The variation in isometric tension with sarcomere length in vertebrate muscle fibres. *J. Physiol.* **184**, 170–192.

Gulbis, J. M. and Doyle, D. A. (2004). Potassium channel structures: do they conform? *Curr. Opin. Struct. Biol.* **14**, 440–446.

Gussak, I. and Antzelevich, C (2003). *Cardiac Repolarization: Bridging Basic and Clinical Science*. Totowa NJ: Humana Press Inc.

Guy, H. R. (1988). A model relating the structure of the sodium channel to its functions. *Curr. Topics Membr. Transp.* **33**, 289–308.

Hamill, O. P., Marty, A., Neher, E., Sakmann, B. and Sigworth, F. J. (1981). Improved patch-clamp techniques for high-resolution current recording from cells and cell-free membrane patches. *Pflügers Arch.* **391**, 85–100.

Hill, A. V. (1938). The heat of shortening and the dynamic constants of muscle. *Proc. R. Soc. Lond.* **B126**, 136–195.

Hill, A. V. (1950a). A challenge to biochemists. *Biochim. Biophys. Acta* **4**, 4–11.

Hill, A. V. (1950b). The dimensions of animals and their muscular dynamics. *Sci. Prog. Lond.* **38**, 209–230.

Hill, A. V. and Hartree, W. (1920). The four phases of heat production of muscle. *J. Physiol.* **54**, 84–128.

Hille, B. (1971). The hydration of sodium ions crossing the nerve membrane. *Proc. Nat. Acad. Sci. USA.* **68**, 280–282.

Hodgkin, A. L. (1939). The relation between conduction velocity and the electrical resistance outside a nerve fibre. *J. Physiol.* **94**, 560–70.

Hodgkin, A. L. (1951). The ionic basis of electrical activity in nerve and muscle. *Biol. Rev.* **26**, 339–409.

Hodgkin, A. L. (1958). Ionic movements and electrical activity in giant nerve fibres. *Proc. R. Soc. Lond.* **B148**, 1–37.

Hodgkin, A. L. (1975). The optimum density of sodium channels in an unmyelinated nerve. *Phil. Trans. R. Soc. Lond.* **B270**, 297–300.

Hodgkin, A. L. and Horowicz, P. (1957). The differential action of hypertonic solutions on the twitch and action potential of a muscle fibre. *J. Physiol.* **136**, 17–18P.

Hodgkin, A. L. and Horowicz, P. (1959). The influence of potassium and chloride ions on the membrane potential of single muscle fibres. *J. Physiol.* **148**, 127–160.

Hodgkin, A. L. and Horowicz, P. (1960). Potassium contractures in single muscle fibres. *J. Physiol.* **153**, 386–403.

Hodgkin, A. L. and Huxley, A. F. (1952). A quantitative description of membrane current and its application to conduction and excitation in nerve. *J. Physiol.* **117**, 500–544.

Hodgkin, A. L., Huxley, A. F. and Katz, B. (1952). Measurement of current voltage relations in the membrane of the giant axon of *Loligo*. *J. Physiol.* **116**, 424–448.

Hodgkin, A. L. and Katz, B. (1949). The effects of sodium ions on the electrical activity of the giant axon of the squid. *J. Physiol.* **108**, 37–77.

Hodgkin, A. L. and Keynes, R. D. (1955a). Active transport of cations in giant axons from, Sepia and Loligo. *J. Physiol.* **128**, 28–60.

Hodgkin, A. L. and Keynes, R. D. (1955b). The potassium permeability of a giant nerve fibre. *J. Physiol.* **128**, 61–88.

Hoffman B.F. and Cranefield, P.F. (1960). *Electrophysiology of the Heart*. New York: McGrawHill.

Homsher, E. (1987). Muscle enthalpy production and its relationship to actomyosin ATPase. *Ann. Rev. Physiol.* **49**, 673–690.

Huang, C.L.-H. (1982). Pharmacological separation of charge movement components in frog skeletal muscle. *J. Physiol.* **324**, 375–387.

Huang C. L.-H. (1990). Voltage-dependent block of charge movement components by nifedipine in frog skeletal muscle. *J. Gen. Physiol.* **96**, 535–557.

Huang, C.L.-H. (1994) Charge conservation in intact frog skeletal muscle fibres in gluconate-containing solutions. *J. Physiol.* **474**, 161–171.

Huang, C. L.-H. (1996). Kinetic isoforms of intramembrane charge in intact amphibian striated muscle. *J. Gen. Physiol.* **107**, 515–534.

Huang, C. L.-H. (1998). The influence of caffeine on intramembrane charge movements in intact frog striated muscle. *J. Physiol.* **512**, 707–721.

Huang, C. L.-H. and Peachey, L. D. (1989). The anatomical distribution of voltage-dependent membrane capacitance in frog skeletal muscle fibres. *J. Gen. Physiol.* **93**, 565–584.

Huxley, A. F. and Niedergerke, R. (1954). Structural changes in muscle during contraction. Interference microscopy of living muscle fibres. *Nature* **173**, 971–973.

Huxley, A. F. and Stämpfli, R. (1949). Evidence for saltatory conduction in peripheral myelinated nerve fibres. *J. Physiol.* **108**, 315–339.

Huxley, A. F. and Taylor, R. E. (1958). Local activation of striated muscle fibres. *J. Physiol.* **144**, 426–441.

Huxley, H. E. (1963). Electron microscope studies on the structure of natural and synthetic protein filaments from striated muscle. *J. Mol. Biol.* **7**, 281–308.

Huxley, H. E. (1976). The structural basis of contraction and regulation in skeletal muscle. In *Molecular Basis of Motility*, ed. L. M. G. Heilmeyer Jr, J. C. Ruegg and Th. Wieland. Berlin: Springer-Verlag.

Huxley, H. E. (1990). Sliding filaments and molecular motile systems. *J. Biol. Chem.* **265**, 8347–8350.

Huxley, H. E. and Hanson, J. (1954). Change in the cross-striations of muscle during contraction and stretch and their structural interpretation. *Nature* **173**, 973–976.

Jiang, Y., Lee, A., Chen, J. *et al.* (2003). X-ray structure of a voltage-dependent K+ channel. *Nature* **423**, 33–41.

Kato, G. (1936). On the excitation, conduction, and narcotization of single nerve fibers. *Cold Spr. Harb. Symp. Quant. Biol.* **4**, 202–213.

Katz, B. and Miledi, R. (1965). The measurement of synaptic delay, and the time course of acetylcholine release at the neuromuscular junction. *Proc. R. Soc. Lond. B* **161**, 483–495.

Katz, B. and Miledi, R. (1967). The timing of calcium action during neuromuscular transmission. *J. Physiol.* **189**, 535–544.

Keynes, R. D. (1951). The ionic movements during nervous activity. *J. Physiol.* **114**, 119–150.

Keynes, R. D. (1963). Chloride in the squid giant axon. *J. Physiol.* **169**, 690–705.

Keynes, R. D. (1994). The kinetics of voltage-gated ion channels. *Q. Rev. Biophys.* **27**, 339–434.

Keynes, R. D. and Elinder, F. (1998a). On the slowly rising phase of the sodium gating current in the squid giant axon. *Proc. R. Soc. Lond. B* **265**, 255–262.

Keynes, R. D. and Elinder, F. (1998b). Modelling the activation, opening, inactivation and reopening of the voltage-gated sodium channel. *Proc R. Soc. Lond. B: Biol Sci.* **265**, 263–270.

Keynes, R. D. and Elinder, F. (1999). The screw-helical voltage gating of ion channels. *Proc. R. Soc. Lond. B* **266**, 843–852.

Keynes, R. D. and Lewis, P. R. (1951). The sodium and potassium content of cephalopod nerve fibres. *J. Physiol.* **114**, 151–182.

Keynes, R. D. and Martins-Ferreira, H. (1953). Membrane potentials in the electroplates of the electric eel. *J. Physiol.* **119**, 315–351.

Keynes, R. D. and Meves, H. (1993). Properties of the voltage sensor for the opening and closing of the sodium channels in the squid giant axon. *R. Soc. Lond. B: Biol Sci.* **253**, 61–68.

Keynes, R. D. and Ritchie, J. M. (1984). On the binding of labelled saxitoxin to the squid giant axon. *Proc. R. Soc. Lond. B* **222**, 147–153.

Keynes, R. D. and Rojas, E. (1973). Characteristics of the sodium gating current in the squid giant axon. *J. Physiol.* **233**, 28–30P

Keynes, R. D. and Rojas, E. (1974). Kinetics and steady-state properties of the charged system controlling sodium conductance in the squid giant axon. *J Physiol.* **239**, 393–434.

Killeen, M. J., Sabir, I. N., Grace, A. A. and Huang, C. L.-H. (2008). Dispersions of repolarization and ventricular arrhythmogenesis: lessons from animal models. *Prog. Biophys. Mol. Biol.* **98**, 219–229.

Koeppen, B. M. and Stanton, B. A. (2009). *Berne & Levy: Principles of Physiology*, 6th edn. New York: Mosby, 848pp.

Kovacs, L., Rios, E. and Schneider, M. F. (1979). Calcium transients and intramembrane charge movement in skeletal muscle fibres. *Nature* **279**, 391–396.

Kuffler, S. W. (1980). Slow synaptic responses in the autonomic ganglia and the pursuit of a peptidergic transmitter. *J. Exp. Biol.* **89**, 257–286.

Kuffler, S. W. and Yoshikami, D. (1975). The number of transmitter molecules in a quantum: an estimate from iontophoretic application of acetylcholine at the neuromuscular synapse. *J. Physiol.* **251**, 465–482.

Kyte, J. and Doolittle, R. F. (1982). A simple method for displaying the hydropathic character of a protein. *J. Mol. Biol.* **157**, 105–132.

Lamb, J. F., Ingram, C. G., Johnston, I. A. and Pitman, R. M. (1991). *Essential Physiology*. 3rd edn. Oxford: WileyBlackwell.

Larsson, H. P., Baker, O. S., Dhillon, D. S. and Isacoff, E. Y. (1996). Transmembrane movement of the Shaker K+ channel S4. *Neuron* **16**, 387–397.

Lei, M., Goddard, C., Liu, J. *et al.* (2005). Sinus node dysfunction following targeted disruption of the murine cardiac sodium channel gene, SCN5A. *J. Physiol.* **567**, 387–400.

Levy, M. N., Koeppen, B. M and Stanton, B. A. (2005). *Berne & Levy: Principles of Physiology*, 4th edn. New York: Mosby.

Loewi, O. (1921). Über humorale Übertragbarkeit der Herzner-venwirkung. *Pflügers Arch. Ges. Physiol.* **189**, 239–242.

Makowski, L., Caspar, D. L. D., Phillips, W. C., Baker, T. S. and Goodenough, D. A. (1984). Gap junction structures VI. Variation and conservation in connexon conformation and packing. *Biophys. J.* **45**, 208–218.

Maylie, J., Irving, M., Sizto, N. L. and Chandler, W. K. (1987). Calcium signals recorded from cut frog twitch fibers containing Antipyrylazo III. *J. Gen. Physiol.* **89**, 83–143.

McCleskey, E. W. (1999). Calcium channel permeation: a field in flux. *J. Gen. Physiol.* **113**, 765–772.

Merton, P. A. (1954). Voluntary strength and fatigue. *J. Physiol.* **128**, 553–564.

Merton, P. A., Hill, D. K. and Morton, H. B. (1981). Indirect and direct stimulation of fatigued human muscle. In *Human Muscle Fatigue: Physiological Mechanisms*, ed. R. Porter and J. Whelan, pp. 120–126. London: Pitman Medical.

Neher, E. and Sakmann, B. (1976). Single-channel currents recorded from membrane of denervated frog muscle cells. *Nature* **260**, 799–802.

Nielsen, O. B., de Paoli, F., and Overgaard, K. (2001). Protective effects of lactic acid on force production in rat skeletal muscle. *J. Physiol.* **536**: 161–166.

Noble, D. (1979). *The Initiation of the Heartbeat*, 2nd edn. Oxford: Oxford University Press.

Noda, M., Shimizu, S., Tanabe, T. *et al.* (1984). Primary structure of *Electrophorus electricus* sodium channel deduced from cDNA sequence. *Nature* **312**, 121–127.

Noda, M., Takahashi, H., Tanabe, T. *et al.* (1982). Primary structure of α-subunit precursor of *Torpedo californica* acetylcholine receptor deduced from cDNA sequence. *Nature* **279**, 793–797.

Offer, G. (1974). The molecular basis of muscular contraction. In *Companion to Biochemistry*, ed. A. T. Bull, J. R. Lagnado, J. O. Thomas and K. F. Tipton, pp. 623–671. London: Longman.

Ostrowski, J., Kjelsberg, M. A., Caron, M. G. and Lefkowitz, R. J. (1992). Mutagenesis of the β_2-adrenergic receptor: how structure elucidates function. *Ann. Rev. Pharmacol. Toxicol.* **32**, 167–183.

Padmanabhan, N. and Huang, C. L.-H. (1990). Separation of tubular electrical activity in amphibian skeletal muscle through temperature change. *Exp. Physiol.* **75**, 721–724.

Papadatos, G. A., Wallerstein, P. M. R., Head, C. E. G. *et al.* (2002). Slowed conduction and ventricular tachycardia after targeted disruption of the cardiac sodium channel Scn5a. *Proc. Nat. Acad. Sci.* **99**, 6210–6215.

Peachey, L. D. (1965). The sarcoplasmic reticulum and transverse tubules of the frog's sartorius. *J. Cell Biol.* **25**, 209–232.

Pedersen, T. H, Macdonald, W. A., dePaoli, F. V., Gurung, I. S. and Nielsen, O. B. (2009). Comparison of regulated passive membrane conductance in action potential firing fast and slow-twitch muscle. *J. Gen. Physiol.* **134**, 323–337.

Pedersen, T. H., Nielsen, O. B., Lamb, G. D., and Stephenson, D. G. (2004). Intracellular acidosis enhances the excitability of working muscle. *Science* **305**, 1144–1147.

Porter, K. R. and Palade, G. E. (1957). Studies on the endoplasmic reticulum. III. Its form and distribution in striated muscle cells. *J. Biophys. Biochem. Cytol.* **3**, 269–300.

Rayment, I. and Holden, H. M. (1994). The three-dimensional structure of a molecular motor. *Trends Biochem. Sci.* **19**, 129–134.

Rayment, I., Smith, C. and Yount, R. G. (1996). The active site of myosin. *Ann. Rev. Physiol.* **58**, 671–702.

Rios, E. and Brum, G. (1987). Involvement of dihydropyridine receptors in excitation-contraction coupling in skeletal muscle. *Nature* **325**, 717–720.

Ritchie, J. M. and Rogart, R. B. (1977). The binding of saxitoxin and tetrodotoxin to excitable tissue. *Rev. Physiol. Biochem. Pharmacol.* **79**, 1–50.

Robertson, J. D. (1960). The molecular structure and contact relationships of cell membranes. *Prog. Biophys.* **10**, 343–418.

Rushton, W. A. H. (1933). Lapicque's theory of curarization. *J. Physiol.* **77**, 337–364.

Ryall, R. W. (1979). *Mechanisms of Drug Action on the Nervous System.* Cambridge: Cambridge University Press.

Scher, A. M. (1965). Electrical correlates of the cardiac cycle. In *Physiology and Biophysics*, ed. T. C. Ruch and H. D. Patten. Philadelphia: Saunders, pp. 565–599.

Schmidt-Nielsen, K. (1990). *Animal Physiology*, 4th edn. Cambridge: Cambridge University Press.

Schneider, M.F. and Chandler, W. K. (1973). Voltage-dependent charge in skeletal muscle: a possible step in excitation-contraction coupling. *Nature* **242**, 244–246.

Schwartz, L. M., McCleskey, E. W. and Almers, W. (1985). Dihydropyridine receptors in muscle are voltage-dependent but most are not functional calcium channels. *Nature.* **314**, 747–751.

Sejersted, O. M. and Sjøgård, G. (2000). Dynamics and consequences of potassium shifts in skeletal muscle and heart during exercise. *Physiol. Rev.* **80**, 1411–1481.

Sheikh, S. M., Skepper, J. N., Chawla, S. *et al.* (2001). Normal conduction of surface action potentials in detubulated amphibian skeletal muscle fibres. *J. Physiol.* **535**, 579–590.

Skou, J. C. (1957). The influence of some cations on an adenosine triphosphatase from peripheral nerves. *Biochim. Biophys. Acta* **23**, 394–401.

Skou, J. C. (1998). Nobel Lecture. The identification of the sodium pump. *Biosci Rep.* **18**, 155–169.

Spudich, J. A. (1994). How molecular motors work. *Nature* **372**, 515–518.

Spudich, J. A., Finer, J., Simmons, B. et al. (1995). Myosin structure and function. *Cold Spr. Harb. Symp. Quant. Biol.* **60**, 703–71.

Squire, J. M. (1986). *Muscle: Design, Diversity and Disease.* Menlo Park, California: Benjamin/Cummings.

Stokoe, K. S., Thomas, G., Goddard, C. A. et al. (2007). Effects of flecainide and quinidine on arrhythmogenic properties of Scn5a+/Δ murine hearts modelling long QT syndrome 3. *J. Physiol.* **578**, 69–84.

Takeshima, H., Nishimura, S., Matsumoto, T. et al. (1989). Primary structure and expression from complementary DNA of skeletal muscle ryanodine receptor. *Nature* **339**, 439–445.

Takeuchi, A. and Takeuchi, N. (1959). Active phase of frog's end-plate potential. *J. Neurophysiol.* **22**, 395–411.

Takeuchi, A. and Takeuchi, N. (1960). On the permeability of the end-plate membrane during the action of the transmitter. *J. Physiol.* **154**, 52–67.

Tasaki, I. (1953). *Nervous Transmission.* Springfield, Illinois: Charles C. Thomas.

Unwin, N. (1993). Nicotinic acetylcholine receptor at 9 Å resolution. *J. Mol. Biol.* **229**, 1101–1124.

Unwin, N. (1995). Acetylcholine receptor channel imaged in the open state. *Nature* **373**, 37–43.

Usher-Smith, J. A., Fraser, J. A., Bailey, P. S. J., Griffin J. L., and Huang, C. L-H. (2006a). The influence of intracellular lactate and H+ on cell volume in amphibian skeletal muscle. *J. Physiol.* **573**, 799–818.

Usher-Smith, J. A., Huang, C. L.-H. and Fraser, J. A. (2009). Control of cell volume in skeletal muscle. *Biol Rev Camb Philos Soc.* **84**, 143–159.

Usher-Smith, J. A., Skepper, J. N., Fraser J. A. and Huang, C. L.-H. (2006b). Effect of repetitive stimulation on cell volume and its relationship to membrane potential in amphibian skeletal muscle. *Eur. J. Physiol.* **452**: 231–239.

Weidmann, S. (1956). *Elektrophysiologie der Herzmuskelfaser.* Huber: Berne.

Whittaker, V. P. (1984). The structure and function of cholinergic synaptic vesicles. *Biochem. Soc. Trans.* **12**, 561–576.

Wilkie, D. R. (1968). Heat work and phosphorylcreatine breakdown in muscle. *J. Physiol.* **195**, 157–183.

Wilkie, D. R. (1976). Energy transformation in muscle. In *Molecular Basis of Motility*, ed. L. M. G. Heilmeyer Jr., J. C. Ruegg and Th. Wieland, pp. 69–80. Berlin: Springer-Verlag.

Yang, N., George, A. L. and Horn, R. (1996). Molecular basis of charge movement in voltage-gated sodium channels. *Neuron* **16**, 113–122.

Zhang, F., Wang, L. P., Boyden, E. S. and Deisseroth, K. (2006). Channelrhodopsin-2 and optical control of excitable cells. *Nature Methods.* **3**, 785–792.

Index